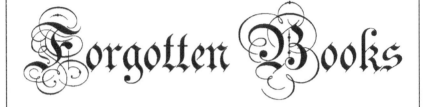

ISBN 978-0-260-23246-5
PIBN 11013589

This book is a reproduction of an important historical work. Forgotten Books uses
state-of-the-art technology to digitally reconstruct the work, preserving the original format
whilst repairing imperfections present in the aged copy. In rare cases, an imperfection in
the original, such as a blemish or missing page, may be replicated in our edition. We do,
however, repair the vast majority of imperfections successfully; any imperfections that
remain are intentionally left to preserve the state of such historical works.

1 MONTH OF
FREE
READING

at
www.ForgottenBooks.com

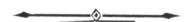

By purchasing this book you are eligible for one month membership to ForgottenBooks.com, giving you unlimited access to our entire collection of over 1,000,000 titles via our web site and mobile apps.

To claim your free month visit:

www.forgottenbooks.com/free1013589

ARISTOTLE'S
MASTER-PIECE,
COMPLETED.
IN TWO PARTS.

The FIRST *containing the Secrets of* GENERATION; *In all the Parts thereof.*

Treating of the benefit of Marriage, and the prejudice of unequal matches. Signs of Insufficiency in men or woman. Of the Infusion of the soul. Of the Likeness of children to parents. Of Monstrous Births. The cause and cure of the Green Sickness. A discourse of Virginity. Directions and cautions for Midwives. Of the Organs of Generation in women, and the fabric of the Womb. The use and action of the Genitals. Signs of Conception, and whether a male or female; with a Word of Advice to both sexes in the act of Copulation. And the Pictures of several Monstrous Births, &c.

The Second Part being a Private
LOOKING GLASS FOR THE FEMALE SEX.

Treating of various Maladies of the Womb, and of all other distempers incident to women of all ages, with proper remedies for the cure of each.

The whole being more correct than any thing of the kind hitherto published.

NEW-YORK:
PRINTED FOR THE COMPANY OF FLYING
STATIONERS. 1807.

INTRODUCTION.

———❦———

IF one of the meanest capacity were asked, 'What 'was the wonder of the world?' I think the most proper answer would be, MAN : he being the little world, to whom all things are subordinate; agreeing in the genius with sensitive things; all, being animals, but differing in the species. For man alone is endowed with reason.

And therefore the Deity, at man's creation (as the inspired penman tells us), said, " Let us make man " in our own immage, that he may be (as a creature " may be) like Us, and the same in his likeness, may " be our immage," Some of the fathers do distinguish as if by the image, the Lord doth plant the reasonable powers of the soul, reason, will and memory; and by likeness the qualities of the mind, charity, justice patience, &c. But Moses confounded this distinction (if you compare these texts of scripture) Gen. i. 17. and v. 1 Coloss. x· Eph. v. 14. And the apostle, where he saith, ' He was created after ' the image of God, knowledge, and the same in ' righteousness and holyness.' The Creeks there represented him as one turning his eyes upwards towards lim, whose image & superscription he bears.

> See how the heav'n's high architect
> Hath fram'd him in this wise,
> To stand to go, to look erect,
> With body, face and eyes.

And Cicero says, like Moses, all creatures were made to rot on the earth, except man, to whom was given an upright frame, to contemplate his Maker, and behold the mansion prepared for him above.

Now, to the end that so noble and glorious a creature might not quite perish, it pleased God to give unto woman the field of generation for a receptacle of human seed, where by that natural and vegitible soul, which lies potentially in the seed, may, by the plastic power, be reduced into act; that man, who is a mortal creature, by leaving his offspring behind him, may become immortal, and survive in his posterity.

And because this field of generation, the womb is the place where this excellent creature is formed, and that in so wonderful a manner, that the Royal Psalmist (haveing meditated thereon) cries out as one in extacy, ' I am fearfully & wonderfully made " It will be necessary to treat largely thereon in this book, which, to that end, is divided into two parts, —the first whereof treats of the manner and parts of generation in both sexes; for, from the mutual desire they have to each other, which nature has implanted into them to that end, that delight which they take in the act of copulation, does the whole race of mankind proceed; and a particular account of what things are previous to that act, and also what are consequential of it, and how each member concerned in it is adapted and fitted to that work, to to which nature has designed it And though in uttering of those things, some thing may be said which those that are unclean may make bad use of, and use it, as a motive to stir up their bestial appetites; yet, such may know that this was never intended for them nor do I know any reason that those sober persons for whose use this was ment, should want the help hereby designed them, because vain, loose persons will be ready to abuse it.

The second part of this tretise is wholly designed for the female sex, and does largely not only treat of the distempers of the womb, and the various causes, but also gives you proper remedies for the cure of them ; for such is the ignorance of most women, that when, by any distemper, those parts are afflicted, they neither know from whence it proceeds, nor how to apply a remedy ; and such is their modesty, also, that they are unwilling to ask, that they may be informed ; and for the help of such this is designed: for having my being from a woman, I thought none had more right to the grapes than she that planted the vine.

And therefore, observing that among all diseases incident to the body, there are none more frequent and perilous than those that do arise from the ill state of the womb; for, through the evil quality thereof, the heart, the liver and the brain are affected, from whence the actions, vital, natural and animal, are hurt, and the virtues concoctive, sanguinificative, distributive, attractive, expulsive, retentive, with the rest, are all weakened ; so that from the womb come convulsions, epilepsies, apoplexies, palsies and fevers, dropsies, malignant ulcers, &c. And there is no disease so bad, but may grow worse from the evil quality of it.

How necessary, therefore, is the knowledge of these things, let every unprejudiced reader judge ; for, that many women labour under them, through their ignorance and modesty (as I said before), woful experience makes manifest : here, therefore (as in a mirror), they may be acquainted with their own distempers, and have suitable remedies, without applying themselves to physicians, against which they have so great reluctance.

ARISTOTLE's
MASTER-PIECE,
COMPLETED.

PART FIRST.

CHAP. I.

Of Marriage, and at what age young men and vir-
gins are capable of it ; and why they so much
desire it : Also, how long men and women are
capable of having children.

THERE are very few, except some professed
debauchees, but what will readily agree, that
marriage is honorable to all, being ordained by heaven in Paradise, and without which no man or woman can be in a capacity honestly to yield obedience
to the first law of the creation—increase and multi-
ply, and since it is natural in young people to desire
these mutual embraces, proper to the marriage bed,
it behoves parents to look after their children, and
when they find them inclinable to marriage, not vi-
olently to restrain their affections, and oppose their
inclinations (which, instead of allaying them, makes
them but the more impetuous) but rather provide.
such suitable matches for them, as may make their
lives comfortable, lest the crossing of their inclinations should precipitate them to commit those follies
that may bring an indelible stain upon their families.

The inclinations of maids to marriage, is to be
known by many symptoms ; for when they arrive at
puberty, which is about the fourteenth or fifteenth
year of their age, then the natural purgations begin
to flow, and the blood, which is no longer taken to
augment their bodies, abounding, stirs up their
minds to venery : External causes also may incite

them to it, for their spirits being brisk and enflamed when they arrive at this age, if they eat hard salt things, and spices, the body becomes more and more heated, whereby the desire to venereal embraces is very great, sometimes almost insuperable. And the use of this so much desired employment being denied to virgins, many times is followed by dismal consequences, as a green wesel colour, short breathings trembling of the heart, &c. But when they are married, and their venereal desires satisfied by the enjoyment of their husbands, those distempers vanish, and they become more gay and lively than before ; also their eager staring at men, and affecting their company, shews that nature pushes them upon coition, and their parents neglecting to get them husbands, they break thro' modesty to satisfy themselves in unlawful embraces ; it is the same in brisk widows, who cannot be satisfied without the benevolence which their husbands used to give them.

At the age of fourteen, the menses in girls begin to flow, when they are capable of conceiving, and continue generally to forty-four, when they cease bearing, unless their bodies are strong and healthful, which sometimes enables them to bear at fifty-five. But, many times the menses proceed from some violence offered to nature, or some morbific matter, which often proves fatal to the party, and therefore those men that are desirous of issue, must marry a woman within the age aforesaid, or blame themselves if they meet with disappointments : Tho' if an old man, not worn out by diseases and incontinency, marry a brisk lively lass, there is hopes of his having children to three score and ten, nay, sometimes till near four score.

Hippocrates holds, that a youth of fifteen years, or between that and seventeen, having much vital strength, is capable of getting children ; and, also, that the force of procreating matter increases till forty-five, fifty, and fifty-five, and then begins to flag, the seeds by degrees becoming unfruitful, the natural spirits being extinguished, and the humours dried up. Thus, in general; but, as to particulars, it often falls out otherwise; nay, it is reported by a credible author, that in Sweden, a man was married at one hundred years, to a bride of thirty, and had many children by her, but his countenance was so fresh, that those that knew him not, took him not to exceed fifty. And in Campania, where the air is clear and temperate, men of 80 years old married young virgins, and had children by them; shewing that age in them hinders not procreation, unless they be exhausted in their youth, and their yards shrivelled up.

If any would know why a woman is sooner barren than a man, they may be assured, that the natural heat, which is the cause of generation, is more predomiuant in the latter than in the former : for, since a woman is truly more moist than a man, as her monthly purgations demonstrate, as also the softness of her body, it is also apparent, that he doth not exceed her in natural heat, which is the chief thing that concocts the humours into proper aliment, which the woman wanting, grows fat; when a man, through his native heat, melts his fat by degrees, and his humours are dissolved, and by the benefit thereof are elaborated into seed. And this may also be added, that woman generally are not so strong as men, nor so wise nor prudent, nor have so much reason and ingenuity in ordering affairs, which shews that thereby their faculties are hindered operations.

CHAP. II.

*How to get a male or female child, and of the embryo
and perfect birth, and the fittest time for copulation.*

WHEN a young couple is married, they naturally desire children, and therefore use
those means that nature has appointed to that end;
but, notwithstanding their endeavours, they must
know that the success of all depends on a blessing of
the Lord; not only so, but the sex, wether male or
female, is from his disposal also; though it cannot
be denied, but secondary causes have influence
therein, especially two,—First the genteial humor,
which is brought by the arteria præ paraentes to
the testes in form of blood, and there elaborated into seed by the seminifical faculty residing in them;
to which may be added, the desire of coition, which
fires the imagination with unusual fancies, and by
the sight of brisk charming beauty, may soon in-
flame the appetite; but if nature be enfeebled, such
meats must be eaten as will conduce to the affording
such aliment as makes the seed abound, and restores
the decays of nature, that the faculties may freely
operate, and remove impediments obstructing the
procreation of children.

Then since diet alters the evil state of the body to
a better, those who are subject to barrenness must
eat such meats as are of good juice, that nourish
well, making the body lively and full of sap, of which
faculty are all hot moist meats: For, according to
Galen, seed is made of pure concocted and windy
superfluity of blood, whence we may conclude there
is a power in many things to accumulate seed, also to augment it, and other things of force to
cause erection, as hen-eggs, pheasants, woodcocks,
gnatsnappers, thrushes, blackbirds, young pigeons,

sprrrows, patridges, capoons, almonds, pine-nuts, raisans, currants all strong wines taken sparingly especially those made of the graps of Italy; but erection is chiefly caused by scuram, eringoes, cresses-crymson, parsnips, artichokes, turnips, rapes, asparagus, candied ginger, galings, acorns bruised to powder drank in muscadel, scallions sea shell fish, &c;— but these must have time to perform their operation, and must use them for a considerable time, or you will reap but little benefit by them. The act of coition being over, let the woman repose herself on her right side with her head lying low, and her body declining, that by sleeping in that posture the cawl on the right side of the matrix may prove the place of the conception, for therein is the greatest generative heat, which is the chief procuring cause of male children, and rarely fails the expectation of those that experience it, especially if they do but keep warm, without much motion, leaning to the right, and drinking a little spirit of saffron & juice of hysop in a glass of Malaga or Alicant, when they lie down & rise, for the space of a week.

For a female child, let a woman lie on the left side, strongly fancying female in the time of procreation, drinking the decotion of female mercury four days from the first day of purgation—the male mercury having the like opperation in case of male, for this concoction purges the right and left side of the womb opens the receptacles, and makes way for the seminary of generation to beget a female the the best time is when the moon is in the wane, in libra or Aquarrius. Advicene says, ' When the menses are spent, and the womb clensed, which is commonly in five or seven days at most, if a man lie with his wife from the first day she is purged to the fifth, she will conceive a male; but from the fifth to the eighth a female; and from the eighth

" to the twelfth a male again ; but after that per-
" haps neither distinctly but both in a heramaphro-
" dite." In a word they that would be happy in the
fruits of their labor, must observe to use copulation
in due distance of time, not too often nor too seldom,
for both are a like hurtful ; and to use it immediatly
weakens and wasts their spirits, and spoils the seed;
and thus much for the particular. The second
is to let the reader know, how the child is formed
in the womb, what accidents it is liable to there,
and how nourished and brought forth.

There are various opinions, concerning this matter therefore I will shew what the learned say about
it. Man consists of an egg, which is impregnated
into the testicles of the woman by the more subtler
part of the man's seed ; but the forming faculty and
virtue in the seed is a divine gift, it being abundant-
ly endued with a vital spirit, which gives sap and
form to the embryo ; so that all parts and bulk of
the body, which is made up in a few months, and
gradually formed into the lovely figure of a man,
do consist in, and are adumbrated thereby, which is
incompareably expressed in the cxxxviii psalm, ' I
" will prase thee O Lord, because i am wonderfully
" made and, &c." And the physicians have slighted
four different times wherein a man is framed and
perfected in the womb, the first moon after coition
being perfect in the first week, if no flux happens,
which sometimes falls out, through the slipperiness
of the matrix of the head thereof, that shifts over
like a rose-bud, and opens on a sudden by means of
forming, is assigned to be when nature makes manifest mutation in the conception, so that all the substance seems congealed flesh and blood, which happens twelve or fourteen days after copulation. And
though this fleshy mass abounds with fiery bloood,
yet it remains undistinguishable, without form of

figure and may be called an embryo, and compared
to seed sown in the ground, which, thro'. heat, and
moisture, grows, by degrees, into a perfect form,
either in plant or grain. The third time assigned
to make up this fabric, is when the principal parts
shew themselves as plain, as the heart, whence proced the arteries. The brain from which the nerves,
like small threads, run through the whole body;
and the liver that divides the chyle from the blood
brought to it by the veny porta, the two first are
fountains of life, that nourish every part of the body,
in fraiming which the faculty of the womb is buried
from the time of conception to the eighth day of
the first month.

  Lastly, about the thirtieth day, the outward parts
are seen finely wrought, and distinguished by joints,
when the child begins to grow, from which time, by
reason the limbs are divided and the whole frame is
perfect, it is no longer an embryo, but a perfect
child. Most males are perfect by the thirtieth day,
but females seldom to the forty-second or forty-fifth
day, because the heat of the womb is greater in producing the male than the female; and for the same
reason, a woman going with a male child quickens
in three months, but going with a female, rarely under four, at which time also its hair and nails come
forth, and the child begins to stir, kick and move in
the womb, and then woman are troubled with loathing of their meet, and greedy longing for things
contrary to nutriment, as coals, rubbish, chalk, &c
which desire often occasions abortion and miscarriage. Some woman have been so extravagant as to
long for hob-nails, leather, men's flesh, horse flesh,
& other unnatural as well as unwholesome food, for
want of which things they have either miscarried,
or the child has continued dead in the womb for several days, to the imminent hazard of their lives.

But I shall now proced to shew by what real means the infant is sustained in the womb, and what posture it there remains in.

Various are the opinions about nourishing the fœtus in the womb : Some say by blood only, from the umbilical vein ; others by the chyle, taken in by the mouth ; but it is nourished diversly according to the several degrees of perfection that an egg passes from a conception to fœtus ready for birth. But, first let us explain the meaning of ovum or the egg : In the generation of the fœtus there are two principals, active and passive—the active is the man's seed elabarated in the testicles, out of arterial blood and animal spirits—the passive is an egg impregnated by the man's seed. And the nature of conception is thus : the most spiritous part of the man's seed in the act of generation, reaching up to the testicles of the woman, which contains diverse ggs, imprignates one of them, which being conveyed by the oviducts to the bottom of the womb, presently begins to swell bigger and bigger, and drinks in the moister that is plentifully sent thither, as seeds suck moisture in the ground, to make them sprout out, when the parts of the embryo begin to be a little more perfect, & that at the same time the chorin is very thick, that the liquor cannot soak thro' it the umbilical vessels begin to be formed and to extend the side of the amnion which they pass thro', and all through the aliantreides and chorin, and are implanted in the placenta, which gathering upon the chorin, joins to the uterus. And now the arteries that before sent out the nourishment into the cavity of the womb, opened by the orifice into the placenta, where they deposit the said juice, which is drank up by the unbilical vein, and conveyed by it, first to the liver of the fœtus, and then to the heart, where its more thin and spiritous part is turned into blood, while the grosser part descending by the aorta, enters the umbilical arteries, and is discharged into its cavity by those branches that run through the aminon.

As soon as the mouth, stomach, gullet, &c. are formed so perfectly, that the fœtus can swallow, it sucks in some of the grosser nutricious juice. that is deposited in the amnion by the umbilical arteries, which descending into the stomach and intestines, is received by the lecteal veins, as in adult persons. The fœtus being perfected, at the time before specified, in all its parts, it lies equally balanced in the womb, as the centre on his head, and being long turned oval, so that the head a little inclines, and it lays its chin upon its breast, its heels and ancles upon its buttocks, its hands on its cheeks, and its thumbs to its eyes; but its legs and thighs are carried upwards, with its hams bending, so that they touch the bottom of its belly, the former and that part of the body which is over against us, as the forehead, nose and face, are towards the mother's back, and the head inclining downwards, towards the rump-bone that joins to the os sacrum, which bone, together with the os pubis, in the time of birth, part is loosed, whence it is, that the male children commonly come with their faces downwards, or with their head turned somewhat oblique, that their faces may be seen, but the female children with their faces upwards; though sometimes it happens that births do not follow according to nature's order, but children come forth with their feet standing, their necks bowed, and their heads lying oblique, with their hands stretched out, which greatly endangers themselves and the mother, giving the midwife great trouble to bring them into the world; but when all things proceed in nature's order, the child when the time of birth is accomplished, is desirous to come forth of the womb, and by inclining himself, he rolls downwards, for he can no more be obscured in those hidden places, and the heat of the heart cannot subsist without external respiration, whereof being grown great more and more desirous of nutriment and light, when covering the ætherial air, by struggling to obtain it, breaks the membranes and coverings, whereby he was restrained and fenced against attrition, and for the most part, with bitter pangs of the mother, issueth forth into the world commonly in the ninth month. For the matrix being divided and the os pubis loosened, the woman strives to cast out her burden, and the child does the like to get forth, by the help of its inbred strength, and so the birth comes to be perfect; but if the child be dead, the more dangerous the delivery, tho' nature often helps the woman's weakness herein ; but the child that is quick and lively, labours no less than the woman.   Now, there are births at seven or eight months, and some women go to the tenth month ; but of these, and the reasons of them I shall speak more largely in another place.

CHAP. III.

The reason why children are like their parents, and that the mother's Imagination contributes thereto, and whether the man or woman is the cause of the male or female child.

LACTANTIUS is of opinion, that when a man's seed falls on the left side of the womb, it may procure a male child; but, because it is the proper place for a female, there will be something in it that resembles a woman ; that is, 'twill be fairer, whiter and smoother, not very subject to have hair on the body or chin ; it will have lank hair on the head, the voice small and sharp, and the cariage feeble and, on the contrary, that a female may chance to be gotten if the seed fall on the right side; but then through the abundance of the heat, she shall be big-boned, full of courage, having a masculine voice, and her chin and bosom hairy, not being so clear as, others of that sex, and subject to quarrel with her husband for superiority.

In case of similitude, nothing is more powerful than the imagination of the mother; for if she fasten her eyes upon any object, and imprint it on her mind, it oftentimes so happens, that the child, in some part or other of its body, has a representation thereof; and if in the act of copulation, the woman earnestly look upon the man, and fix her mind upon him, the child will resemble its father. Nay, tho' a woman in unlawful copulation, yet if she fix her mind upon her husband, the child will resemble him though he never got it. The same effect of imagination causes warts, stains, molth-spots, dastes, tho' indeed they sometimes happen through frights or extravagant longing; many woman being with child, seeing a hare cross them, will, through the force of imagination, bring forth a child with a hare-lip. Some children are born with flat noses, wry 'mouths, great blubber lips, and ill-shaped bodies; and must ascribe the reason to the imagination of the mother, who hath cast her eyes and mind upon some ill-shaped creature; Therefore, it behoves all woman with child, if possible, to avoid such sights or, at least, not regard them. But though the mother's imagination may contribute much to the features of the child, yet in manners, wit and propension of the mind experience tells us, that children are commonly of the condition with the parents, and same tempers But the vigour or disability of persons in the act of copulation, many times causes it to be otherwise; For children got thro' the heat

and strength of desire, must needs partake more of
the nature and inclination of their parents, than
those that are begotten with desires more week:
And, therefore, the children begotten by men in
their old age, are generally weaker than those begotten by them in their youth.

As to the share which each of the parents has in
begetting the child, we will give the oppinion of the
ancients about it.

Though it is apparant (say they) that the man's
seed if the chief efficient beginning of action, motion
and generation : yet, that the woman affords seed,
and effectually contributes in that point to the procreation of the child is evinced by strong reasons.
In the first place, seminary vessels have been given
her in vain, and genital testicles inverted, if the woman wanted seminal exscrescence ; for nature doth
nothing in vain ; therefore, we must grant they were
made for the use of seed, and procreation, and fixed
in their proper place both the testicles and receptacles of seed, whose nature is to opperate and afford
virtue to the seed. And to prove this, their needs
no stronger argument (say they) than, that if a woman do not use copulation, to eject her seed, she often falls into strange diseases, as appear by young
women & virgins : A second reason they urge, is,
that although the society of a lawful bed consist not
altogether in these things, yet it is apparant, the
female sex are never better pleased, nor appear
more blith and jocund then when they are satisfied
this way ; which is an inducement to believe, they
have more pleasure & titillation therein than men.
for, since nature, causes much delight to company
ejection, by the breaking forth of the swelling spirits and the sweetness of the nerves, in which case
the opperation on the woman's part is double, she

having an enjoyment both by ejection and reception, by which she is more delighted in the act.

. Hence it is (say they), that the child more frequently resembles the mother than the father, because the mother contributes most towards it. And they think it may be further instanced, from the endeared affection they bare to them ; for that besides contributing seminal matter, they feed and nourish the child with the purest fountain of blood, until its birth. Which opinion Galen affirms, by allowing children to partisipate most of the mother, and ascribes the differance of sex to the operation of the menstrual blood ; but the reason of the likeness, he refers to the power of the seed; for as plants receive more nourishment from fruitful ground than from the industry of the husbandman, so the infant receieves in more abundance from the mother than the father. For, first, the seed of both is cherished in the womb, and there grows to perfection, being nourished with blood : and for this reason it is (say they) that children for the most part, love their mother best, because they receive most of their substance from their mother : For about nine months she nourishes her child in her womb, with her purest blood ; then, her love towards it, newly born, and its likeness, do clearly shew, that the woman affordeth seed and contributes more towards making the child than the man.

. But, in all this the ancients are very erronious, for the testicles (so called in woman) afford not any seed, but are two eggs, like those of fowls, and other creatures ; neither have they any office as those of men but are indeed ovaria, wherein the eggs are nourished by the sanguinary vessels dispersed through them ; and from hence one or more (as they are fecundated by the man's seed) is separated, and conveyed into the womb by the oviducts.

—The truth of this is my plan, for, if you boil them, their liquor will be the same colour, tast and consistencey with the taste of birds eggs. If any object, they have no taste that signifies nothing ; for the eggs of fowls, while they are in the ovary, nay, after they are fastened to the uterus, have no shell : And though, when they are laid, they have one, yet' that is no more than a defence which nature has provided them against any outward injury, while they are' hatched without the body ; whereas those, of the woman being hatched within the body, need no other defence than the womb, by which they are sufficiently secured.

And this is enough, I hope for the clearing of this point. As to the third thing proposed, as whence grows the kind and whether the man or woman is the cause of the male or female infant ?

The primary cause we may ascribe to God, as is, most justly his due who is the ruler&disposer of all things, yet he suffers many thing to proceed according to the rules of nature, which proceed by their inbred motion, according to usual and natural courses without variation. Tho', indeed by favour from on high, Sarah conceived Isaac—Hannah, Samuel—& Elizabeth, John the Baptist : But these are all very extraordinary things, brought to pass by a Divine Power, above the course of nature ; nor have such instances been wanting in latter days, therefore I shall wave them and proceed to speak of things natural. The ancient physicians and philosophers say, that since that there are two principals out of which the body of man is made, and which renders the child like his parents, and by one or the other sex, viz. seed, common to both sexes, and menstrual blood, propper to the woman only, the similitude (say they) must needs consist in the force of virtue of the male or female, so that it proves

like the one or the other according to the plenty af-
forded by either.; but that the differance of the sex
is not referred to the seed, but to the menstrual
blood, which is proper to the woman, is apparent.
For were that force altogether retained in the seed;
the male seed being of the hottest quality male chil-
cren would abound, and few of the females be propagated ; wherefore, the sex is atributed to the temperament of the active qualities, which consist in
the heat and cold and the nature of the matter under
them ; that is the flowing of the menstrous blood ;
but now the seed (say they) affords both force to
procreate & form the child, and matter for its generation . and in the menstruous blood there is both
matter and force ; for, as the seed most helps the
material principal, so also does the menstrual blood
the potential seed ; which is (says Galen) blood
well concocted by the vessels that contain it. So
that blood is not only the matter for genrating the
child, but all seed in possibility that menstrual
blood hath both principals.

The ancients further say, that the seed is the
stronger efficient ; the matter of it being very little
in quality but the potential quality of it is very
strong ; whereof, if these principals of generation,
according to which the sex is made, where only
(say they) in the menstrual blood then would the
children be all mostly females ; as, where the efficient force in the seed, they would be all males ;
but since both have opperation in menstrual blood,
matter predominates in quantity ; and in the seed,
force and virtue. and therefore Galen thinks the
child receives its sex rather from the mother than
from the father; for, tho' his seed contributes a little
to the material principal yet it is more weekly. But
for likeness, it is refered rather to the faher than
to the mother. Yet the woman's seed receiving

strength from the menstrual blood, for the space of nine months, overpowers the man's as to that particular; for, the menstrual blood flowing in the vessels rather cherishes the one than the other; from which it is plain, the woman affords both matter to make, and force and virtue to perfect the conception; though the female's seed be fit nutriment for the male's, by reason of the thinness of it, being more adapted to make up conception thereby. For as of soft wax and moist clay, the artificer can frame what he intends, so (say they) the man's seed mixing with the woman's, and also with the menstrual blood, helps to form and perfect part of man.

But with all imaginable deference to the wisdom of our fathers, give me leave to say, that their ignorance in the anatomy of man's body, has led them into the paths of error, and run them into great mistakes; for their hypothesis of the formation of the embryo from the coto-mixture of seed, and the nourishment of it, too, in the menstruous blood, being wholly false, their opinion, in this case, must, of necessity, be so also.

I shall, therefore, conclude this chapter, and only say, that, altho' a strong imagination of the mother may often determin the sex, yet the main agent in this case is the plastic and formative principal, which is the efficient in giving form to the child, which gives this or that sex, according to those laws and rules given to us by the wise Creator of all Things, who both makes and fashions it, and therein determines the sex, according to the counsel of his own will.

CHAP. IV.

*A discourse of Man's Soul, that it is not propaga-
ted by the parents; but is infused by the Creator,
and can neither die nor corrupt. At what time
it is infused. Of its Immortality, aud certainty
of the resurrection.*

MAN's soul is of so divine a nature and ex-
cellency, that man himself cannot, in any
wise, comprehend it, it being the infused breath of
the Almighty, of an immortal nature, and not to be
comprehended but by him that gave it. For, Moses, by holy inspiration, relating the original of
man, tells us, "that God breathed into his nostrils
" the breath of life, and he became a living soul."
Now, as for all other creaturs, at his word they
were made, and had life. but the creatur God had
appointed to set over his works, was the peculiar
workmanship of the Almighty, forming him out of
the dust of the earth, and condescending to breathe
into his nostrils the breath of life, which seems to
denote more care and (if we may so term it) labour.
used about man. than about all others creaturs, he
only partaking and participating of the blessed divine nature, bearing God's image in innocence and
purity, whilst he stood firm, and when, by his fall,
that lively image was defaced, yet such was the
love of his Creator towards him, that he found out a
way to restore him—the only-begotten Son of the
Eternal Father coming into the world to destroy
the works of the Devil, and to raise up Man from
that low condition to which his sin and fall had reduced him, to a state above that of angels.

If, therefore, man would understand the excel-
lency of his soul, let him turn his eyes inwardly &
look into himself, and search diligently his own
mind, and there he shall see many admirable gifts

C

and excellent ornaments that must needs possess
him with wonder and amazement, as reason, understanding freedom of will, &c. that plainly shew the
soul to be descended from a heavenly original, and
that, therefore, it is of infinite duration, and not subject to annihilation. Yet, for its many offices and operations whilst in the body, it goes under several de-
nomminations ; For, when it enlivens the body, it is
called the soul ; when it gives knowledge, the judgment or mind ; and when it recals things past, the
memory, whilst it discourses and discerns, reason ;
whilst it contemplates, the spirit ; whilst it is the
sensitive parts, the senses. And these are the principal offices, whereby the soul declares its power,
and performs its action ; for, being seated in the
highest parts of the body, it diffuseth its force into
every member ; not propagated from the parents,
nor mixed with gross matter, but the infused breath
of god immediately proceeding from him, not passing from one to another, as was the opinion of Py-
thagoras, who held a transmigration of the soul,
but that the soul is given to every infant by infusion, is the most received and orthodox opinion ; and
the learned do likewise agree, that this is done when
the infant is perfected in the womb, which happens
about the twenty-fourth day after conception, esp-
cially for males, who are generally born at the end
of nine months ; but in females, who are not so soon
formed and perfected, thro' defect of heat not till
the fiftieth day. And though this day, in all cases,
cannot be truly set down, yet Hypocrates has given
his opinion, when the child has its perfect form,
when it begins to move, and when born, if in due
season. In his book of the nature of infants he says,
if it be a female, and he be perfect on the thirtieth
day, and move on the ninetieth day, he will be born

on the seventh month; but if he be perfectly formed on the thirty-fifth day, he will move on the seventieth and be born on the eighth month; again, if he be perfectly formed on the fifty-fifth day, he will move on the ninetieth, and be born on the ninth month. Now from those passing of days and months it plainly appears, that the day of forming being doubled, makes up the day of moving, and that day three times reckoned, makes up the day of birth. .

As thus, when thirty-five perfects the form, if you double it, makes seventy, the day of motion, and three times seventy amount to two hundred and ten days, which, allowing thirty days to a month, makes seven months; and so you must consider the rest. But, as to a female, the case is different; for, it is longer perfecting in the womb, the mother ever going longer with a boy than a girl, which makes the account differ; for, a female formed in thirty days, moves not till the seventieth day, and is born in the eighth month: when she is formed on the fortieth, she moves not till the eightieth, and is born on the eighth month; but, if she be perfectly formed on the fifty-fifth day, she moves on the ninetieth, and is born on the ninth month; but, if she that is formed on the sixtieth day, moves the hundred-and-tenth, and will be born on the tenth month. I treat the more largely hereof, that the ready may know, the reasonable soul is not propagated by the parents; but is infused by the Almighty, when the child hath its perfect form, and is exactly distinguished in its lineaments.

Now, as the life of every other creature, as Moses shews, is in the blood, so the life of man consisteth in the soul, which, although subject to passion, by reason of the gross composures of the body, in which it has a temporary confinement, yet it is immortal and cannot in itself corrupt or suffer change,. it being a spark of the Divine Mind ; and that eve-ry man has a peculiar soul, plainly appears by the difference between the will, judgement, opinion, manners and affections in men. And this David ob-serves, saying, " God hath formed the hearts and " minds of all men, and hath given to every one his " own being and a soul of its own nature." Hence, Solomon rejoiced that God had given him a happy soul and a body agreeable to it. It has been dispu-ted among the learned in what part of the body the soul resides ; aud some are of opinion, its residence, is in the middle of the heart; and from thence com-municates itself to every part, which Solomon, in Proverbs iv. seems to affirm, when he says, ' Keep ' thy heart with all diligence, for out of it are the ' issues of life.' But many curious physicians, searching the works of nature in man's anatomy, do affirm that its chief seat is, in the brain, from whence proceeds the senses, faculties and actions, diffusing the operation of the soul thro' all the parts. of the body whereby it is enlightened with heat and force to the heart, by the arteries, corditcs, or slee-. py arteries, which part upon the throat, the which,. if they happen to be broken or cut, they cause barrenness ; and if stopped, an apoplexy ; for, there must necessarily be ways thro' which the spirits, animal and vital, may have intercourse, and convey native heat from the soul. For, though the soul hath its chief seat in one place, it operates in every part, exercising every member which are the souls instruments by which she discovers her pow-er. But if it happens that any of the organical parts are out of tune, its whole work is confused, as appears in ideots & madmen, tho' in some of them the soul, by vigorous exerting its power recovers its innate strength, and they become right after a long despondency in mind; but in others it is not recovered again in this life. For as a fire under ashes, or the sun obscured from our sight by thick clouds, afford not their full lustre, so the soul overwhelmed in moist or morbic matter,is darkened, & reason overclouded; and though reason shines less in children than such as are arrived to maturity, yet no man must imagine that the soul of an infant grows up with the child,for then would it again decay; but it suits itself to nature's weakness, and the imbecility of the body wherein it is placed that it may opperate the better. And as the body is more and more capable of receiving its influence, so the soul does more and more exert its faculties, having force and endowments at the time it enters the form of a child in the womb, for its substance can receive nothing less. And thus much to prove the soul comes not from the parents, but is infused by God. I shall next prove its immortality, and so demonstrate the certainty of our resurrection.

That the soul of man is a divine ray, infused by the Sovereign Creator, I have already proved; and now come to shew that whatever immediately proceeds from him, and participates of his nature, must be as immortal as its origin; for, though all other creatures are endowed with life and motion, yet they want a reasonable soul; and from thence it is concluded, that their life is in their blood, and that being corruptible they perish and are no more; but man being endowed with a reasonable soul, & stamped with the divine image, is of a different nature; and tho' his body be corruptible, yet his soul being of an immortal nature, cannot perish, but must, at the dissolution of his body, return to God who gave it, either to receive reward, or punishment. Now, that the body can sin of itself is

C 2

impossible; because, wanting the soul, which is
the principal of life, it cannot act, nor proceed to
any thing either good or evil; for, could it do so,
it might sin even in the grave; but it is plain, that
after death there is a cessation; for, as death
leaves us, so judgement will find us.

Now, reason having evidently demonstrated the
soul's immortality, the holy scriptures do abud-
antly give testimony to the truth of the resurrection, as the reader may see by perusing the 9th
and 14th chapters of Job, and the 5th of St. John,
I shall, therefore, leave the further discoursing of
this matter to divines, whose proper province it is,
and return to treat of the works of nature.

CHAP. V.

Of Monsters, and Monstrous Births.

MONSTERS are properly depraved conceptions, and are deemed by the ancients to be excur-
sions of nature, and are always vicious, either in
figure, situation, magnitude or number.

They are vicious in figure, when a man bears the
character of a beast; they are vicious in magnitude,
when the parts are not equal, or that one part is bigger than the other; and this is a thing very-com-
mon, by reason of some excrescence. They are vicious in situation many ways, as if the ears were on
the face, or the eyes on the breasts or on the legs,
as was seen in a monster born at Ravenna in Italy,
in the year 1570. And, lastly, they are vicious in
number, when a man hath two heads, four hands,
and two bodies joined, which was the case of the
monster born at Zazara in the year 1550.

As to the cause of their generation, it is either
divine or natural The divine cause proceeds from
the permissive will of the great Auther of our being, suffering parents to bring forth such depraved

monsters, as a punishment for their filthy and corrupt affections, which are let loos unto wickedness
like brute beasts that have no understanding; for
which reason the ancient Romans enacted, that'
those who were deformed should not be put into
religious houses. And St. Jerome, in his time,
grieved to see the deformed and lame offered up
to God in religious houses; and Kecherman, by
way of inference, excluded all that were mishapen,
because outward deformity of body is often a sign
of the pollution of the heart, being a curse laid upon the child for the incontinence of the parents. Yet
there are many born deformed, which deformed
ought not to be ascribed to the parents. Let us therefore search out the natural cause of their generation, which, according to the ancients, who have
dived into the secrets of nature, is either in the
matter of the agent, in the seed, or in the womb.
The matter may be in fault two ways, either by defect or by excess; by defect, when the child hath
but one arm or one leg, &e. by excess, when it
has three hands or two heads. Some monsters are
also begotten by woman's bistial and unatural coition, &c. The agent or womb may be in fault three
ways; First, In the forming faculty, which may be
too strong or two weak; by which a deprived
figure is sometimes produced: Secondly, the instrument or place of conception; the evil con-
formation or evil disposition whereof will cause a
monstrous birth. And, Thirdly, the imaginative
power at the time of conception, which is of such
force that it stamps a character of the thing ima-
gined upon the child; so that the child or the
children of an adulteress, by the mother's imaginative power, may have the nearest resemblance to
her own husband, though begotten by any other
man. And thor' this power or imaginative faculty

it was, that a woman, at the time of conception, be-
holding the picture of a blackamoor, conceived and
brought forth a child, resembling an' Ethiopian.
And that this power of imagination was well enough know to the ancients, is evident by the example of Jacob, the father of the twelve tribes of
Israel, who having agreed with his father-in-law
to have all the spotted sheep for the keeping of
his flock, to increase his wages, took hazel-rods,
pealing them with white streaks in them, and laid
them before the sheep when they came to drink,
and they coupling together, whilst they beheld the
rods, concieved and brought forth spotted young.
Nor does the imagination work on the child at the
time of conception only, but afterwards also ; as
was seen in the example of a worthy gentlewoman, who being big with child, and passing by a
butcher killing meat, a drop of blood sprinkled on
her face; whereupon she presently said that the
child would have some blemish on its face, which
proved true, for at the birth it was found marked
with a red spot.

But besides the way already mentioned, monsters are sometimes produced by other means : to
wit, by the undue coition of a man and his wife
when her monthly courses are upon her ; which
being a thing against nature, no wonder that it
should produce an unnatural issue. If therefore
a man's desire be ever so great for coition, (as
sometimes it is after long absence.) yet if a woman
knows that the custom of women is upon her, she
ought not to admit of any embraces, which at that
time are both unclean and unatural· The issue
of these unclean embraces proving often monstrous, as a just punishment for such a turpidinous
action. Or if they should not always produce

monstrous births, yet are the children thus begotten for the most part dull, heavy, sluggish, and defective in the understanding, wanting the vivacity and liveliness which those children who are begotten when woman are free from their courses are endued with.

Therehas been some contending among authors, to know whether those who are born monsters have reasonable souls, some affirming, and others denying it, the result of both at last coming to this, that those who, according to the order. of nature, are descended from our first parents by the coition of a man and a woman, though their outward shape be deformed and monstrous, have notwithstanding reasonable souls; but those monsters that are not begotten by man, but are the product of a woman's unatural lust, and copulating with other creatures, shall perish as the brute beasts by whom they were begotten, not having a reasonable soul. The same being also true of imperfect and abortive births.

There are some of opinion that monsters may be engendered by infernal spirits; but notwithstanding Ægidius Facius pretended to believe it with respect to a deformed monster born at Cracovia; & Hieronimus writeth of a maid that was got with child by the devil; but he being a wicked spirit, and not capable of having human seed, how is it possible he should beget a human creature? If they say the devil may assume to himself a dead body and enliven the faculties of it, and thereby make it able to generate; I answer, that though we suppose this could be done, which I believe not, yet that body must bear the image of the devil; and it borders upon blasphemy to think, that the all-wise and good Being would so far give way to the worst of spirits, as to suffer him to raise up his diabolical offspring: for in the school of nature we are taught the contrary, vz, that like begets like, whence it follows, that a man cannot be begot of a devil.

The first I shall present is a most frightful monster indeed, representing an hairy child. It was covered over with hair like a beast. But what rendered it yet more frightful was, that its navel was in the place where his nose should stand, and his eyes placed where his mouth should have been, and its mouth was in the chin. It was of the male kind, and born in France, in the year 1597; of which the following is a figure.

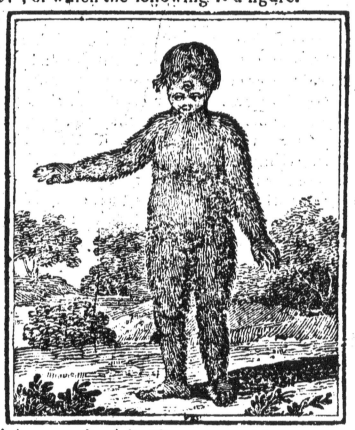

A boy was born in Germany with one head and one body; but having four ears, four arms;

four thighs, four legs, and four feet. This birth
the learned, who beheld it, judged to proceed from
the redundance of the seed: but there not being
enough for twins, nature formed what she could,
and so made the most of it. This child lived
some years, and though he had four feet, he knew
not how to go :—by which we may see the wisdom of nature, or rather the goodness of nature,
and of natur's God, in the formation of the body
of man. See the annexed figure.

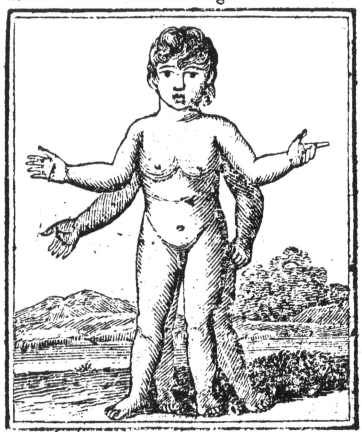

Heaven in our first formation did provide
Two arms, two legs : but what we have beside
Renders us monstrous and mishapen too,
Nor have we any work for them to do;
Two arms, two legs, are all that we can use,
And to have more there's no wiseman will chuse.

In the time of king Henry III. a woman was
delivered of a child, having two heads and four
arms, and the rest was a twin under the navel; and
then beneath all the rest was single, as appears in
the plate below.   The heads were so placed that
they looked contrary ways, and each had two distinct arms and hands: they would both laugh,
both speak, and both cry, and eat and be hungry
together.   Sometimes the one would speak, and
the other keep silence, and sometimes both would
speak together.   It was of the female sex, and
though it had two mouths, and did eat with both,
yet there was but one fundament to disburden
nature.   It lived several years, but the one out.

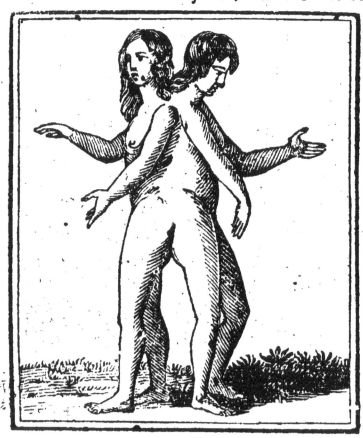

lived the other three years, carrying the dead one (for there was no parting them) till the other fainted with the burden, and more with the sink of the dead carcase.

A child was born in Flanders which had two heads and four arms, seeming like two girls joined together, having two of their arms lifted up between and above their heads; the thighs being placed as it were across one another, according to the figure in the following plate. How long they lived I had no account of.

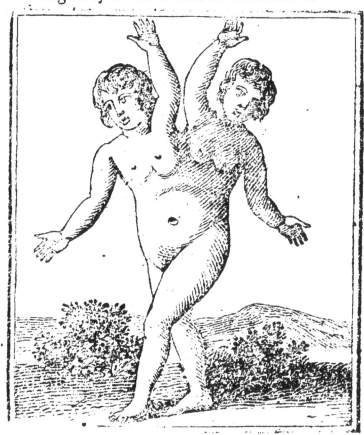

Nature to us does sometimes monsters show,
That we by them may our own mercies know;
And thereby sin's deformity may see,
Than which there's nothing can more monstrous be

D

CHAP. VI.

*A discourse of the happy state of Matrimony, as it is
appointed of God, and the true felicity that re-
dounds thereby to either sex, and to what end it is
ordered.*

WITHOUT doubt, the uniting of hearts in
holy wedlock is of all conditions the hap-
piest, for then a man has a second self, to whom
he can unravel his thoughts, as well as a sweet companion in his labour ; he has one in whose breast, as
in a safe cabinet, he may repose his inmost secrets, especially where reciprocal love and inviolate
faith is settled ; for there no care, fear, jealousy,
mistrust on hatred can ever interpose. For what
man ever hated his own flesh, and truly a wife, if
rightly considered, as our grandfather observed,
is or ought to be esteemed of every honest man,
bone of his bone, and flesh of his flesh, &c. Nor
was it the least care of the Almighty to ordain so
near an union, and that for two causes, the first
for increase of posterity, the second to bridle and
bind man's wandering desires and affections ; nay,
that they might be yet happier when God had
joined them together, he blessed them, as it is in
the ii. of Genesis.   Columily contemplating this
happy state, tells out of the Economy of Xeno-
phon, that the marriage bed is not only the most
pleasant, but profitable course of life that may be
entered on for the preservation and increase of
posterity ; wherefore since marriage is the most
safe, sure, and delightful station of mankind, who
is exceeding prone, by the dictates of nature, to
propagate his like, he does in no ways provide

amiss for his own tranquility who enters into it, especially when he comes to maturity of years, for there are many abuses in marriage, contrary to what is ordained, which in the ensuing chapter I shall expose to view.

But to proceed, seeing our blessed Saviour and his holy apostles detested unlawful lust and pronounced those to be excluded the kingdom of heaven, that poluted themselves with adultry and whoring. I cannot conceive what face persons can have to colour their impieties, who, hating matrimony. make it their study how they may live licentiously; but in so doing, they rather seek to themselves torment, anxiety and disquietudes, than certain pleasure. besides the hazard of their immortal soul ; for certain it is, mercenary love, or (as the wise man calls them) harlots smiles, cannot be true and sincere, & therefore not pleasant, but rather a net laid to betray such as trust in them into all mischief as Solomon observes, by the young men void of understanding, who turned aside to the harlot's house. As a bird to the snare of the fowler, or an ox to the slaughter, till the dart be struck through the liver. Nor in this case can they have children, those endearing pledges of conjugal affection ; or if they have. they will rather redound to their shame than comfort, bearing the odious brand of bastards : Harlots, likewise, are like swallows flying in the summer season of prosperity, but the black stormy weather of adversity coming. they take wings and fly into other regions ; that is, seek themselves other lovers, but a virtuous chaste wile, fixing her entire love upon her husband, and submitting to him

as her head and king, by whose directions she
ought to steer in all lawful courses, will, like a
faithful companion, share patiently with him in
adversities, run with cheerfulness through all difficulties and dangers, though ever so hazardous,
to preserve or assist him in poverty. sickness, or
whatever other misfortune may befal him ; acting
according to her duty in all things ; but a proud,
imperious harlot will do more than she lists in the
sun shine of prosperity ; and like a horse-leech,
ever craving and never satisfied, still seeming dis-
pleased if all her extravagant cravings be not
answered, not regarding the ruin and misery she
brings upon him by those means, though she
seems to dote upon him. uisng to confirm her hy-
pocrisy with crocodile's tears, vows and swoonings,
when her cully is to depart awhile, or seems but
to deny her immoderate desires; yet this lasts no
longer than she can gratify her appetite and prey
upon his fortune. Remarkable is the story that
Cornadus, Gosmer tells us of a young man trav-
elling from Athens to Thebes who met by the way
a beautiful. lady ; as to appearance she seemed
adorned with all perfection of beauty, glittering
with gould and precious stones. This seemed
fair one saluted him, and inviting him to her
house, not far off, pretending to be exceedingly
enamoured with him, and declared she had a long
time waited for an opportunity to find him alone,
that she might reveal her passion to him. The
young spark went with her. and when he came to
her house, he found it, to appearance, built very
stally, and very well furnished; which so far
wrought upon his covetous inclination, that he re-

solved to put off his intended journey, and yield
to her enticements; but whilst she was leading
him to see the pleasant places adjoining to the
house, came up a holy pilgrim, who seeing in
what danger the youth was, resolved to set him in
his right senses and shew him what he amagin-
ed real, was quite otherways; so that by powerful
prayer the mist was taken from before his eyes,
who then beheld his lady ugly, deformed, and
monstrous, and that whatever had appeared glorious and butiful, was only trash. Then he made
her confess what she was, and her design upon
the yong man, which she did, saying, She was
one of the Lamiœ or Faries, and that she had
thus enchanted him on purpose to get him into
her power, that she might devour him. This
passage may be fully alluded to harlots, who draw
those that follow their misguiding lights into the
place of danger, till they have caused them to
shipwrack their fortune, and then leave them to
struggle with the storms of adversity which they
have raised. Now on the contrary, a loving,
chaste and even-tempered wife, seeks what she
may to prevent such dangers, and in every condition does all to make him easy. And, in a word,
as there is no content in the embraces of a harlot, so there is no greater joy than in the reciprocal affection and endearing embraces of a
loving, obedient and chaste wife. Nor is that the
principal end for which matrimony was ordained,
but that the man might follow the law of his creation, by the increasing of his kind, and replenish
the earth, for this was the injunction laid upon
him in Paradise before his fall.——To conclude, a
virtuous wife is a crown and ornament to her hus-
hand, and her price is above rubies; but the ways

CHAP. VII.

*Of errors in Marriage, why they are, and the Pre-
judice of them.*

BY errors in marriage, I mean the unfitness of
the persons marrying to enter into this
state, and that both with respect to age and the
constitution of their bodies ; and therefore those
that design to enter into that condition ought to
observe their ability, and not run themselves upon inconveniencies ; for those that marry too
young, may be said to marry unseasonably, not
considering their inability, nor examining the
force of nature ; for though some, before they
are ripe for consummation of so weighty a matter, who either rashly of their own accord, or by
the iustigation of procurers of marriage-brokers,
or else forced thereto by their parents, who co-
vet a large dowry, take upon them this yoke to
their prejudice. by which some, before the expi-
ration of a year, have been so enfeebled, that all
their vital moisture has been exhausted, which
hath not been restored again without great trouble and the use of medicines. Wherefore my
advice is, that it is no ways convenient to suffer
children, or such as are not of age, to marry or
get children ; but he that proposes to marry, must
observe to chuse a wife of an honest stock, descended of temperate parents, being chast, well
bred, of good manners. For, if a woman have
good conditions, she hath portion enough. That
of Almenian in Plutus, is much to the purpose,
where he brings in a young woman speaking.

" I take not that to be my dowry, which
    The vulgar sort do wealth ,and honor call,

But all my wishes terminates in this,
   To obey my husband and be chaste withal;
To have God's fear and beauty on my mind,
   To do those good who're virtuously inclind'd."
And I think she was in the right of it, for such a
wife is more precious that rubies.

It is certainly the duty of parents to be careful
in bringing up their children in the ways of
virtue, and to have regard to their honor and
reputation, and especially of virgins, when grown
to be marriageable. For, as has been before
noted, if through the too much severity of parents, they may be crossed in their love, many
of them throw themselves into the unchaste arms
of the next alluring tempter that comes in the
way, being, through the softness and flexibility
of their nature, and the strong desire they have
after what nature strongly incites them to, essily
induced to believe man's false vows of promised
marriage, to cover their shame, and then too
late their parents repent of their severity, which
has brought an undeliable stain upon their
families.

Another error in marriage is, the inequality
of years in the parties married; such as for a
young man, who, to advance his fortune, marries
a woman old enough to be his grandmother, between whom, for the most part, strife, jealousies,
and discontent, are all the blessings which crown
the genial bed, it being impossible for such to
have any children. The like may be said, tho'
with less excuse, when an old doating fellow
marries a virgin in the prime of youth and vigor,
who, while he strives to please her, is thereby

wedded to his grave. For, as in green youth it is
unfit and unseasonable to think of marriage, so
to marry in old age is. altogether the same; for
they that enter upon it too soon are soon exhausted, and fall into consumptions and divers
other diseases, and those that procrastinate and
marry unseemly, fall into the like inconveniencies; on the other side, having only this honor,
of an old man they become young cuckolds, especially if their wives have not been trained up in
the paths of virtue, and lie too much open to the
importunity and temptation of lude and debauch-
ed men. Aud thus for the errors of rash, incon-
siderate and inconsiderable marriages.

CHAP. VIII.

*The Opinion of the Learned concerning children, con-
ceived and born within Seven months, with argu-
ments upon the Subject, to prevent suspicion of Incontinency, and bitter contests on that account:
To which are, added, Rules to know the desposi-
tion of Man's Body by the Genital parts.*

MANY bitter quarrels happen between men
and their wives, upon the mans supposition
that his child came to soon, and by consequence
that he should not be the father ; where as it was
through want of understanding the secrets of nature, that brought the man into that error ; and
which had he known, might have cured him of
his suspicion and jealousy ; to remove which, I
shall endeavor to prove that it is possible, and has
been frequently known, that children have been
born at seven months. The cases of this nature
that have happened, have made work for lawyers,
who have left it to physicians to judge by view-

ing the child weather it be a child in seven, eight, or ten months.——Paul, the councellor. has this passage, in the nineteenth book of pleading, viz. It is now a received truth, that a perfect child may be born in the seventh month, by the authority of the learned Hypocrates, and therefore we must believe that a child born at the end of the seventh month in lawful matrimony, may be lawfully begotted. Galen is of opinion that there is no certain time set for bearing of children; and that from Pliny's authority, who makes mention of a woman that went thirteen months with child, but as to what concerns the seventh month, a learned author said—I know several married people in Holland, that had twins born in the seventh month, who lived to old age, having lusty bodies, and lively minds, Wherefore their opinion is absurd, who assert that a child at seven months canno tbe perfect and long lived; and that he cannot, in all parts be perfect till the ninth month, thereupon 'this author proceeds to tell a passage from his own knowledge, viz. Of late says he, there happened a great disturbance among us, which ended not without bloodshed, and was occasioned by a virgin whose chastity had been violated, descended of a noted family, of unspotted fame. Now several charged the fact upon the judge, who was president of a city in Flanders, who stifly denied it, saying, he was ready to take his oath that he never had any carnal copulation with her, that he would not farther that which was none of his. And farther argued, that he verily believed that it was a childborn in seven months, himself being

many miles distant from the mother of it when
it was conceived, whereupon the judges decreed,
that the child should be viewed by able physicians,
and experienced women, & that they should make .
their report; who having made diligent enquiry,
all of them of one mind, concluded the child (without respecting who was the father) was born within the space of seven months, and that it was carried in the mothers womb but twenty-seven weeks
and odd days; but if she should have gone full nine
months, the child's parts and limbs would have
been more firm and strong, & the structure of the
body more compact, for the skin was very loose,
and the breast-bone that defends the heart. and
the gristle that lay over the stomach lay higher
than naturally they should be ; not plain, but crooked and sharp ridged, or pointed like those of a
young chicken, hatched in the beginning of spring.
And being a female, infant it wanted nails upon the
joints of the fingers, upon which, from the mascu-
lous, or cartilaginous matter of the skin, nails that
are very smooth to come, and by degrees harden,
she had instead of nails a thin skin or film. As for
her toes, there was no sign of nails upon them,
wanting the heat which was expanded to the fingers, from the nearness of the heart.   All this being considered, and above all, one gentlewoman of
quality that assisted, affirming that she had been
the mother of nineteen children, and that divers
of them had been born and lived at seven months ;
they, without favour to any party, made their report, that the infant was a child of seven months,
though within the seventh month, for in such cases, the revolution of the moon ought to be observ-

ed, which perfects itself in four bare weeks, or
somewhat less than twenty-eight days, in which
space of the revolution, the blood being agitated
by the force of the moon, ought the courses of the
woman to flow from them, which being spent, and
the matrix being cleansed from the menstruous
blood, which happens on the forth day, then 'if a
man on the seventh day lie with his wife, the copulation is most natural, and then is the conception
best, and the child thus begotten may be born in
the seventh month, and prove very healthful ; So
that upon this report the supposed father was pronounced innocent, upon proof that he was one hundred miles distant all that month in which the
child was begotten; and as for the mother, she
strongly denied that she knew the father, being
forced in the dark, and so through fear and surpize
was left in ignorance.

As for coition, it ought not to be had unless the
parties be in health, lest it turn to the disadvan-
tage of the children so begotten, creating in them
thro' the abundance of ill humors, divers lan-
guishing diseases, wherefore health is no way better to be discerned than by the genitals of the man.
For which reason midwives, and other skilful women, where formerly wont to see the testicles of
children, thereby to conjecture their temperture
and state of the body ; and young men may know
thereby the signs or symptoms of death ; for if the
cases of the testicals be loose & feeble,& the cods fall
down it denots, that the vital spirits, which are the
props of life, are fallen ; but if the secret parts be
wrinkled and raised up it is a sign all is well ;
but that the event may exactly answer the perdic-

.tion, it is necessary to consider what part of the body the disease·possesseth; for if it chance to be the upper part that is afflicted, as the head or stomach, then it will not so well appear by the members, which are unconcerned with such grievances; but the lower part of the body exactly sympathizing with them their liveliness on the contrary makes it apparent; for nature's force, and the spirits that have their intercourse, first manifest themselves therein, which occasion midwives to feel the genitals of children, to know in what part the grief is resided, and whether life or death be portended thereby, the symptoms being strongly communicated by the vessels, that have their intercourse with the principal seat of life.

CHAP. IX.

Of the Green Sickness in Virgins, with its Causes, Signs, and Cures; together with the chief occasion of Barreness of Woman, and the means to remove the Cause, and render them Fruitful:

THE Green Sickness is so common a distemper in Virgins especially those of phlegmatic complexion, that it is easily discerned shewing itself by discoulering the face, making it look green, pale and of a dusty couler: preceding from raw and indigested humours; nor doth it only appear to the eye, but sensibly afflicts the person, with difficulties of breathings, pains in the head, palpitations of the heart, with unusual breathings, and small throbbings of the arteries in the temples, neck, and back, which often casts them into fevers, when the humour is over vicious; also loathing of meat, & the distension of the hypochondican part, by reason of the inordinant effluction of the menstrous blood to the greater vessels; and, from the abundance of humours, the whole body Is often troubled with swelling, or at least the thighs, legs, and ancles, all above the heels. There is also a great weariness of the body, without any reason for it.

The Galenical physicians affirm, that this distemper proceeds from the womb, occasioned by the abundance of gross, vicious and rude humours arising from several inward causes; but there are, also, outward causes, which have a share in the production of it; as taken cold in the feet, drinking of water, intemperance of diet, eating of things contrary to nature, viz. raw or burned flesh, ashes, coals, old shoes, chalk, wax, nut-shells, mortar, line, oat-meal, tobacco-pipes, &c. which occasion both a suppression of the menses, and obstructions through the whole body; therefore, the first thing necessary to vindicate the cause is matrimonial conjunction, and such copulation as may prove satisfactory to her that is afflicted; for, then the menses will begin to flow, according to their natural and due course, and the humours being dispersed, will soon waste themselves; and then no more matter being admited to increase them, they will vanish, and a good temperament of body will return; put, in case this best remedy cannot be had soon enough, then blood her in the ancles; and if she be about the age of sixteen, you may likewise do it in the arm, but let her blood but sparingly especially if the blood be good. If the disease be of

E

any continuance, then it is to be eradicated by purging, preparation of the humour first considered, which may be done by the virgin's drinking decoct of guiacam, with dittanyofCreete: but the best purge in this case ought to be made of aloes, agric, senna, rhubarb; and for strengthening the bowels and opening obstructions, chalybeat medicines are chiefly to be used. The diet must be moderate, and sharp things by all means avoided. And for binding the humours, take prepared steel, bezoar stone, the root of sconzonera, oil of chrystal in small wine, and let the diet be moderate but in no wise let vinegar be used therewith nor upon any occasion. And in so observing, the humours will be dilated and dispersed, whereby the complexion will return, and the body be lively and full of vigour.

And now, since barrenness daily creates discontent, and that discontent breeds difference between man and wife, or, by immediate grief, frequently casts the women into one or other distemper, I shall in the next place treat thereof.

OF BARRENNESS.

Formerly, before woman came to the marriagebed, they were first serched by the midwife, and those only which she allowed of as fruitful were admitted. I hope, therefore, it will not be amiss to shew you how they may prove themselves, and turn the barren ground into a fruitful soil. Barrenness is a deprivation of life and power, which ought to be in seed, to procreate and propagate—for which end men and women were made;

Causes of Barrenness.——It is caused by overmuch cold or heat, driving up the seed, and corrupting it, which extinguishes the life of the seed.

making it waterish, and unfit for generation.—It may be caused also by not flowing, or overflowing of the courses, by swelling, ulcers, and inflammations of the womb, by an excrescence of flesh growing about the matrix, by the mouth of the womb being turned to the back or side, by fatness of the body, whereby the mouth of the matrix is closed up, being pressed with the omentum or cawl, and the matter of the seed is turned too fat; or, if she be of a lean and dry body, to the world, she proves barren; because, though she doth conceive, yet the fruit of her body will wither before it comes to perfection, for want of nourishment.— Silvius ascribes one cause of barrenness to compelled copulation: as when parents force their daughters to have husbands contrary to their liking, therein marrying their bodies and not their hearts, and where there is a want of love, there, for the most part, is no conception, as very often appears in women which are deflowered against their wills. Another main cause of this barrenness is attributed to want of a convenient moderating quality which the woman ought to have with the man; as, if he be hot, she must be cold; if he be dry, she must be moist; but if they be both dry, or both moist of constitution, they cannot, propagate;' and yet, simply considered of themselves, they are not barren; for he and she, who were before as the barren fig-tree, being joined to an apt constitution, become as the fruitful vine. And, that a man and woman being every way of like constitution, cannot procreate, I will bring nature itself for a testimony, who hath made man of the better constitution than woman, that the quality of the one may moderate the quality of the other.

Signs of Barrenness.

If barrenness doth procede from over-much heat, she is of a dry body, subject to anger, hath black hair, quick pulse, her purgations flow but little and that with pain, she loves to play in the courts of Venus. But if it comes by cold, then are the signs contrary to those even now recited. If through the evil quality of the womb, make a suflumigation of red storax, myrrh, cassia wood, nutmeg, and cinnamond, and lether recieve the fume of it into the womb, covering her very close ; and if the odour so recieved, passeth through the body up into the mouth and nostrils, of herself she is fruitful ; but if she feals not the fume in her mouth and nose, it argues barrenness one of these ways, that the spirit of the seed is either through cold extinguished, or through heat disipated; If any woman be suspected to be unfruitful, cast natural brimstone, such as are digged out of the mine, in her urin and if worms breed therein, of herself she is not barren,

PROGNOSTICS.

Barrenness makes woman look young, because they are free from those pains and sorrows which other woman are accustomed to bring forth withall.—Yet they have not the full perfection of health which fruitful woman do enjoy ; because they are not rightly purged of the menstrous blood and superflous seed which two are the principal causes of most uterine diseases.

CURE-

First the cause must be removed, and the womb

strengthened, and the spirits of the seed enlivened.

If the womb be over-hot, take surrup of succory with rhubarb, syrup of violets endive, roses, cassia, and purslain. Take of endive, water-lillies, borage flowers, of each a handful ; rhubarb, mirobalan, of of each three drams ; with water make a decoction, and to the straining of the syrup, electuary of violets one ounce, syrup of cassia half an ounce, manna three drams ; make a potion. Take of syrup of mugwart one ounce, syrup of maidenhare two ounces ; puly, elect, triansand one dram, make a julep. Take pru. salut, elect. ros. measure of each three drams, rhubarb one scruple, and make a bolus, apply to the reins and privities fomentations of the juice of lettice, violet roses, mallows, vine-leaves and nightshade ; anoint the secret parts with the cooling unguent of Galen.

If the power of the seed be extinguished by cold take every morning two spoonfuls of cinnamond water, with one scruple of mythridate : Take syrup of calamint, mugwort betony, of each one ounce ; water of penny-royal, feverfew, hysop, sage, of each two ounces, make a julep : Take oil of aniseed two scrupels and a half, diaciminia, diacliathi, diamosci, diaglaangae, of each one ounce, sugar four ounces of water of cinnamond, make lozenges, and take of them a dram and a half twice a day, two hours before meals ; fasten cupping glasses to the hips and belly Take of styrax of caliment, one ounce ; mastic cinnamon, light, aloes, and frankincense, of each half an ounce, musk ten grains, ambergrease half a scrupel, with rose water make a confection, divide it into four equal parts, of one part make a pomum odoratum to smell on, if she be not hysterical; of the second make a mass of pills and let her take three every night; of the third make a pessary dip it in the oil of spikenard, and put it up; of the fourth make a suffumigation for the womb.

If the faculties of the womb be weakened, and the life of the seed suffocated by over much humidity flowing to these parts, Take of betony, marjoram, mugwort penny-royal. balm of each a handful, roots of allom, fennel of each two drams, aniseed, cumming of each one dram, with sugar and water a sufficient quantity, make a syrup, and take three ounces every morning.

If barrenness proced from dryness, consuming the matter of the seed—take every day almond-milk, and goat's milk extracted with honey. But often of the root satyron candied, and of the electuary of diasyron. Take three wedders' heads boil them until the flesh comes from the bones, then take meliot, violets, camomile mercury, orchis with their roots, of each a handful feenigreek, lint seed valerian roots, of each one pound let those be decocted in the aforesaid broth, and let the woman sit in the decoction, up to the navel.

If barrenness be caused by any proper effect of the womb, the cure is set down in the second part; sometimes the womb proves barren when there is no impediment on either side except only the manner of the act as when iu the emision of the seed, the man is quick and the womsn too slow, whereby there is not any emision of both seeds at the same instant as the rules of conception requires before the acts of coition, foment the private parts with the decoction of betony, sage, hysop, and calamint; and anoint the mouth and neck of the womb with musk and civet.

The cause of barrenness being removed, let the womb be corroborated as follows:

Take of bay-berries, mastic nutmeg, frankin-sance, nuts, laudanum, gaipunum, of each one dram, styrasis liquid two scrupels, cloves half a scrupel ambergrese two grains, then with oil of spikenard make a pessary.

The aptest time for conception is instantly after the mensis are ceased, because then the womb is thursty and dry, apt to draw the seed and return it by the roughtness of the inward superfi-cies. And beside in some the mouth of the womb is turned into the back or side, and is not placed right until the day of the courses.

Excess in all things is to be avoided; lay aside all passion of the mind, shun, study and care, as things that are enemies to conception; for if a woman conceives under such circumstances, how wise soever the parents are, the children, at best, will be but foolish, because the animal faculties of the parents, viz. the understanding and the rest (from whence the child derives its reason) are, as it were, confused, through the muitiplicity of cares and cogitations; examples hereof we have in learn-ed men, who after great study and care, instantly accompany wiih their wives, often beget very fool-ish children. A hot and moist air is convenient, as appears by the woman of Egypt, who usually bring forth three or four children at one time.

CHAP. X.

*Virginity, what it is, in what it consists, and how
violated ; together with the Opinion of the Learned about the Mutation of the Sex in the Womb, during the Operation of Nature in framing the Body.*

THERE are many ignorant people that boast of
their skill in their knowledge of virginity,
and some virgins have undergone hard censures
through their ignorant determinations ; and, therefore,I thought it highly necessary to clear this point,
that the towering imaginations of conceited ignorance may be brought down,and the fair sex (whose
virtues are so illustriously bright, that they both
excite our wonder, and command our imitation)
may be freed from the calumnies and detractions
of ignorance and envy ; and so their honours may
continue as unspotted as they have kept their persons uncontaminated, and free from defilement.

Virginity, in a strict sense, does signify the
prime, the chief, the best of any thing, which
make men so desirous of marrying virgins, ima-
gining some secret pleasure to be enjoyed in their
embraces, more than in those of widows, or such as
before hath been laid withal, though not many years
ago, a very great person was of another mind, and
to use his own expressions, " that the getting of a
" maiden head was such a piece of drudgery,as was
" more proper for a porter than a prince." But
this was only his opinion, for most men, I am sure,
have other sentiments. But to our purpose.

The curious inquirer's into nature's secrets have
observed, that in young maids, in the sinu pudoris,
or in that place which is called the neck of the
womb, is that pondous production vulgarly called

the hymen, but more rightly the claustrum virginale, and in the French, " button de rose," or rose bud, because it resembles the bud of a rose expanded, of a conve gilly-flower. From hence is derived the word defloro, or deflower. And hence taking away virginity is called deflowering a virgin. Most being of opinion, that the virginity is altogether lost when this duplication is fractured and dissipated by violence ; and when it is found perfect and entire, no penetration has been made ; and it is the opinion of some learned physicians, that there is not either hymen or skin expanded, containing blood in it, which divers think in the first copulation flows from the fractured expanse.

Now, this claustrum virginale, or flower, is composed of four carbuncles or little buds, like myrtle-berries, which in virgins are full and plump, but in women flag and hang loose ; and these are placed in the four angles of the sinus pudoris joined together by little membranes and ligatures like fibres, each of them situated in the testicles, or spaces between each carbuncle, with which, in a manner, they are proportionably distended, which membranes being once delacerated, denote devirgination ; and many inquisitive, and yet ignorant persons, finding their wives defective herein the first night of their marriage, have thereupon suspected their chastity, and concluded another had been there before them. Now, to undeceive such, I do affirm, that such fractures happen divers accidental ways, as well as by copulation with men, viz. by violent straining, coughing, sneezing, stopping of urine, and violent motion of the vessels forcibly sending down the humours, which pressing for passage, break the ligatures or membrane ; so that the intireness of fracture of that which is commonly taken for their virginity or maiden-head, is not an absolute sign of dishonesty ; though, certain it is, that it is more frequently broke in copulation than by any other means.

I have heard, that at an assize held at Rutland, a young man was tried for a rape, in forcing a virgin ; when, after divers questions asked, and the maid swearing positively to the matter, naming the time, place, and manner of the action ; it was, upon mature deliberation, resolved, that she should be-searched by a skilful surgeon and two mid-wives, who were to make their report upon their oaths : which, after due examination, they accordingly did, affirming, that the membrane were entire, and not delacerated ; and that it was their opinion, for that reason, that her body had not been penetrated. Which so far wrought with the jury, that the prisoner was acquitted ; and the maid afterwards confessed, she swore against him out of revenge, he having promised to marry her, and afterwards declined it. And this much shall suffice to be spoken concerning virginity.

I shall now proceed to something of nature's operation in mutation of sexes in the womb.

This point is of much necessity, by reason of the different opinions of men relating to it , therefore, before any thing positively can be asserted, it will be altogether convenient to recite what has been delivered, as well in the negative as affirmative. And, first, Severus Plinus, who argues for the negative, writes thus :—The genital parts of both sexes are so unlike others in substance, com-

position, situation, figure, action, and use, that nothing is more unlike; and by how much more all
parts of the body (the breasts accepted, which in
women swell more, because nature ordained them
for suckling the infant) have exact resemblance; so
much more do the genital parts of the one sex compared with the other differ: and if their figure be
thus different, much more in their use. The venereal appetite also proceeds from different causes;
for in man it proceeds from a desire of emission,
and in woman from a desire of reception; in women, also, the chief of those parts are concave, and
apt to receive; but in men they are more porous.

These things considered, I cannot but wonder
(added he) how any one can imagine that the genital members of the female births should be
changed unto those that belong to males; since by
those parts only the distinction of sexes is made;
nor can I well impute the reason of this vulgar error to any thing, but the mistake of unexpert midwives, who have been deceived by the evil confor-
mation of the parts, which in some male births
may have happened to have some small protrusions,
not to have been discerned; as appears by the example of a child christened at Paris by the name
of Joan as a girl, which afterwards proved a boy;
and, on the contrary, the over-far extension of the
clytoris in female births, may have occasioned the
like mistakes.—Thus far Pliny proceeds in the
negative; And yet notwithstanding what he has
said, there are divers learned physicians that have
asserted the affirmative, of which number Galen is
one. A man (saith he) is different from a woman
in nothing else but having his genital members

without the body ; but a woman hath them within. It is certain, that if nature having formed, should convert him into a woman ; she hath no other task to perform, but to turn his genital members inward, and so turn a woman into a man by the contrary operation, but this is to be understood of the child when it is in the womb, and not perfectly formed ; for, divers times nature hath made a female, and it hath so remained in the womb of the mother for near a month or two, and afterward, plenty of heat increasing in the genital members, they have issued forth, and the child has become a male, yet retaining some certain gestures unbefitting the masculine sex ; as female actions, a shrill voice, and a more effeminate temper than ordinary ; contrary-wise, nature having often made a male, and cold humours flowing to it, the genitals being inverted, yet still retaining a masculine air both in voice and gestures. Now, though both these opinions are supported by several reasons, yet I esteem the latter more agreeable to truth ; for, their is not that vast difference between the genitals of the two sexes, as Pliny would have us to believe there is ; for, a woman has, in a manner, the same members with the man, tho' they appear not outward, but are inverted, for the conveniency of generation ; the chief difference being, that the one is solid, and the other porous ; and the principal reason for changing sexes is, and must be attributed to heat or cold, suddenly and slowly contracted, which operates according to its greater or lesser force.

CHAP. XI.

*Directions and Cautions for Midwives, and how
first a Midwife ought to be qualified.*

A MIDWIFE that would acquit herself well in
her employment, ought by no means to enter upon it rashly or unadvisedly, but with great
caution, considering that she is accountable for all
the mischief that befalls through her wilful ignorance or neglect ; therefore, let none take upon
them the office barely upon pretence of maturity
of years and child bearing, for in such, for the
most part, there are divers things wanting that
ought to be observed, which is the occasion so many women and children are lost. Now, for a midwife, in relation to her person, these things ought
to be observed, viz. She must neither be too young
nor too old, neither extraordinary fat, nor weakened by leanness ; but in a good habit of body ;
not subject to diseases, fears nor sudden frights ;
her body well-shaped, and neat in her attire ; her
hands smooth and small ; her nails ever pared
short, not suffering any rings to be upon her finger
during the time she is doing her office, nor any
thing upon her wrists that may obstruct. And to
these ought to be added activity, and a convenient
strength, with much cautiousness and diligence ;
not subject to drowsiness, nor apt to be impatient.

As for her manners, she ought to be courteous,
affable, sober, chaste, and not subject to passion,
bountiful and compassionate to the poor, and not
covetous when she attends upon the rich.

Her temper chearful and pleasant, that she may
the better comfort her patient in the dolorous la-

F

bors; nor must she at any time make too much haste, though her business should require her in another case, lest she thereby endanger the mother of the child.

Of spirit, she ought to be wary, prudent, and cunning; but above all, the fear of God ought to have the ascendant in her soul, which will give her both knowledge and discretion, as the Wise Man tells us.

CHAP. XII.

Further Directions for Midwives, teaching them what they ought to do, and what to avoid.

SINCE the office of a midwife has so great an influence on the well or ill-doing of women and children—in the first place, let her be advantageous to her practice, never thinking herself so perfect but that she may add to her knowledge by study and experience; yet, never let her make an experiment at her patient's cost, nor apply any experiment in that case, unless she has tried them, or knows they will do no harm; practising neither upon poor nor rich, but speaking freely what she knows, and by no means prescribing such medicines as will cause abortion, though desired; which is a high degree of wickedness, and may be termed murder. If she be sent for to them she knows not, let her be very cautious ere she goes, lest by laying an infectious woman, she endanger the spoiling of others, as sometimes it happens; neither must she make her house a receptacle for great-bellied women to discharge their burdens in, lest her house get an ill name, and she thereby lose her practice.

In laying of women, if the birth happen to be large and difficult, she must not seem to be concerned, but must cheer up the woman, and do what she can to make her labour easy. For which she may find directions in the second part of this book.

She must never think of any thing but doing well, causing all things to be in readiness that are proper for the work, and the strengthening of the woman, and receiving the child; and above all let her take care to keep the woman from being unruly when her throes are coming upon her, lest she thereby endanger her own life and the child's.

She must also take care she be not too hasty in her business but wait God's leisure for the birth; and by no means let her suffer herself to be disordered by fear, though things should not go well, lest it should make her incapable of giving that assistance which the labouring woman stands in need of; for, when we are most at a loss, then there is most need of prudence to set things right.

And now, because she can never be a skilful midwife that knows nothing but what is to be seen outwardly, I shall not think it amiss, but, on the contrary, highly necessary, with modesty to describe the generative parts of women, as they have been anatomized by the learned, and shew the use of such vessels as contribute to generation.

CHAP. XIII.

Of the Genitals of Women, external and internal, to the Vessels of the Womb.

IF it were not for public benefit, especially of the practitioners and professors of the art of

midwifery, I would forbear to treat of the secrets
of nature, because they may be turned, by some
lascivious, and lewd persons into ridicule. But
they being absolutely necessary to be known in
order to public good, I will not omit them, because some may make a wrong use of them.
Those parts that offer themselves to view at the
bottom of the belly, are the fissura magnaor,
great chink, with its labia or lips, the mons veneris, and the hair ; these are called by the general
name pudenda, from shame-facedness, because
when they are bare, they bring pudor or shame
upon a woman. The fissura magna reaches from
the lower part of the os pubis to within an inch
of the anus, but it is lesser and closer in maids
than in those that have borne children ; and has
two lips, which, towards the pupis, grow thicker
and more full ; and meeting upon the middle of
the os pupis, makes that rising hill that is called
mons veneris, or the hill of Venus.

The next thing that offers are, the nympha and
clytoris, the former of which is of a membrany
and flammy substance, spungy, soft, and partly
fleshy, and of a red colour, in the shape of wings,
two in number, though, from their rise, they are
placed in an acute angle, producing there a fleshy
substance, which clothe the clytoris ; and sometimes they spread so far, that incision is required
to make way for the man's instrument of generation.

The clytoris is a substance in the upper part of
the division where the two wings concur, and is
the seat of venereal pleasure, being like a yard in

situation; substances composition and erection; growing sometimes out of the body two inches, but that never happens unless through extreme lust, or extraordinary accidents. This clytoris consists of two spungy and skinny bodies, containing a distinct original from the os pubis, the head of it being covered with a tender skin, having a hole or passage like the penis or yard of a man; though not quite through, in which, and the bigness, it only differs from it.

'The next things are fleshy knobs, and the great neck of the womb; and these knobs are behind the wings, being four in number, and resemble myrtle-berries, being placed quadrangular, one against the other; and in this place inserted to the orifice of the bladder, which opens itself into the fissures, to evacuate the urine; for securing of which from the cold, or the like inconveniency, one of these knobs is placed before it, and shuts up the passage.

The lips of the womb, that next appear, being separated, disclose the neck thereof, and in the two things are to be observed, which is the neck itself, and the hymen, but more properly the claustrum virginale, of which before I have discours. ed. By the neck of the womb is to be understood the channel that is between the aforesaid knobs and the inner bone of the womb, which receives the penis like a sheath; and that it may the better be dilated for the pleasure of procreation, the substance of it is sinewy, and a little spongy; and in this concavity are divers folds, or obicular plaits made up tunicles, wrinkled like an expanded rose.

In virgins they plainly appear, but in women that
have often used copulation, they are extinguished; so that the inner side of the womb's neck appears smooth, and in old women it appears more
hard and gristled.   But though this channel be
at sometimes wreathed and crooked; sinking
down, yet, in the time of copulation, labour, or
the monthly purgations, it is erected and extended, which over-extensions occasion the pains of
child-birth.

The hymen, or clanstrum virginale, is that
which closes the neck of the womb, being, as I
have fore-cited in the chapter relating to virginity,
broken in the first copulation, its use being rather
to stay the untimely courses in virgins, than to
any other end; and commonly, when broken in
copulation, or by any other accident, a small
quantity of blood flows from it, attended with
some little pain.   From whence some observe,
that between the duplicity of the two tunicles,
which constitute the neck of the womb, there are
many veins and arteries running along and arising from the vessels on both sides of the thigh,
and so passing into the neck of the womb, being
very large, and the reason thereof is, for that the
neck of the bladder requires to be filled with abundance of spirits, thereby to be dilated for its better taking hold of the penis, there being great
heat required in such motions, which become
more intense by the act. of frication, and consumes a considerable quantity of moisture, in the
supply of which large vessels are altogether necessary.

Another cause of the longr less of these vessels
is, by reason the menses mak e their way through
them, which often occasions women with child to
continue their purgation, for though the womb be
shut up, yet the passage in th e neck of the womb
through which the vessels pa ss, are open: In this
case there is further to be ob served, that as soon
as you penetrate the pudend am, there appear two
little pits or holes wherein is contained an humour,
which being expunged in th e time of copulation,
greatly delights the woman.

CHAP. XIV.

*A Description of the Womb's Fabric, the preparing
Vessels, and Testicles in Women ; as also of the
Difference and ejaculatory Vessels.*

IN the lower part of the hypogastrium, where the
lips are widest and broadest, they being greater
and borader thereabout than those of men, for
which reason they have likewise broader buttocks
than men, the womb is joined to its neck, and is
p aced between the bladder and strait gut, which
keeps it from swaying or rowling, yet gives it
liberty to stretch and dilate itself again to contract,
nature in that case disposing it. Its figure is in
a manner round, and not uulike a gourd, lessening
a little and growing more acute towards one end,
being knit together by its proper ligaments; its
neck likewise is joined by its own substance and
certain membranes that fasten unto the os sacrum,
and the share bone. As to its largeness that much
differs in women, especially the difference is great
between such as have borne children, and those
that have borne none. In substance it is so thick
that it exceeds a thimble breadth, which after

copulation is so far from decreasing, that it aug-
ments to a greater proportion, and the more to
strengthen it, it is interwoven with fibres over-
thwart, which are both straight and winding, and
its proper vessels are veins, arteries and nerves,
and among these there are two little veins which
pass from the spermatick vessels to the bottom of
the womb, and two larger from the hypostratic,
which touch both the bottom of the neck, the
mouth of these veins, piercing as far as the inward
concavity.

The womb hath two arteries on both sides the
spermatick vessels and the hypostratic, which will
accompany the veins; and besides there are divers
little nerves, that are knit and twined in the form
of a net, which are also extended throughout, even
from the bottom of the pudenda, themselves being placed chiefly for sense and pleasure, moving
in sympathy between the head and the womb.

Now it is to be further noted, that by reason of
the two ligaments that hang on either side the
womb from the share bone, piercing through the
pritoneum, and joined to the bone itself, the womb
is moveable upon sundry occasions, often falling
low or rising high. As for the neck of the womb,
it is of an exquisite feeling, so that if it be at any
time out of order, being troubled at any time with
a schirrosity, over-fatness, moisture, or relaxation,
the womb is subjected thereby to barrenness; in
those that are with child there frequently stays a
glutinous matter in the entrance to facilitate the
birth; for at the time of delivery, the mouth of
the womb is opened to such a wideness as is con-
formable to the bigness of the child, suffering an
equal dilation from the bottom to the top.

As for the preparatory or spermatic vessels in women, they consist of two veins and two arteries not differing from those of men, but only of their largeness and manner of insertion, for the number of veins and arteries is the same as in men; the right vein issuing from the trunk of the hollow vein descending, and on the side of them are two arteries, which grow from the aorta.

As to the length and breadth of these vessels they are narrower and shorter in women than in men; only observe, they are more wreathed and comforted than in men, as shrinking together by reason of their shortness, that they may, by their looseness, be better stretched out when occasion requires it; and those vessels in women are carried with an indirect course through the lesser guts, the testicles, but are in midway divided into two branches, the greater goes to the stones, constituting a various or winding body, and wonderfully inosculating, the lesser branch ending in the womb, in the inside of which it dispers eth itself, and especially at the higher part of the bottom of the womb for its nourishment, and that part of the courses may purge through the vessels; and s..e in the testicles of women are seated near the womb for that cause these vessels fall not from the peritonæum, neither make they much passage as in men, nor extending themselves in the share bone,

The stones in women commonly called testicles, perform not the same action as in men, they are also different in their location, bigness, temperature, substance, form and covering. As for the place of their seat, it is in the hollowness of the abdomen; neither are they pendulous, but rest upon the muscles of the loins, so that they may, by contracting the greater heat, be more fruitful, their office being

to contain the ova or eggs, one of which being impregnated by the man's seed engenders man, yet
they differ from those of men in figure, by reason
of their lessness or flatness at each end, not being
so round or oval. The external superfices being
likewise, more unequal, appearing like the composition of a great many knobs and kernels mixt together. There is a difference also in their substance, they being much more soft and pliable,
loose and not so well compacted.

Their bigness and temperament being likewise
different, for they are much colder and lesser than
those in men. As for their covering or inclosure,
it differs extremely; for as mens are wrapped in
divers tunicles, by reason they are extremely pendulous, and subject to divers injuries, unless so
fenced by nature; so women's stones, being internal, and less subject to casualty, are covered
with one tunicle or membrane, which though it
closely cleave to them, yet they are likewise half
covered with peritonœum.

The ejaculatory vessels are two obscure passages, one on each side, nothing differing from
the spermatick veins in substance: They do rise
on one part, from the bottom of the womb, not
reaching from the other extremity, either to the
stones, or to any other part, but shut up and un-
passable, adhering to the womb as the colon does
to the blind gut, and winding half way about:
though the testicles are remote to them, and touch
them not yet they are tied to them by certain membranes resembling the wing of a bat, through which
certain veins and arteries passing through the end
of the testicles, may be turned here to have their
passages proceeding from the corner of the womb
to the testicles, and are accounted proper liga-

ments, by which the testicles and the womb are uni-
ted, and strongly kint together; and those ligaments
in women are the cremasters in men : of which
i shall speak more largely, when I come to describe the masculine parts, conducing to generation.

CHAP. XV.

*A description of the use and action of several parts
in Woman, appointed in Generation.*

THE externals, commonly called the penden-
da, are designed to cover the great orifice,
and that are to receive the penis or yard, in the act
of coition, and give passage to the birth and urine.
The use of the wings and knobs like myrtle-berries, are for the security of the internal parts, shut-
ting the orifice and neck of the bladder, and by their
swelling up, cause titulation and delight in those
parts, and also to obstruct the voluntary passage
of the urine.

The action of the clytoris in women, is like that
of a penis in man, viz. the erection, and its outer end
like that of the glans of the penis, and has the same
name. And as the glans of man is the seat of the
greatest pleasure in conception, so is this in women.

The action and use of the neck of the womb is
equal with that of the penis, viz. erection, occasioned divers ways, first in copulation it is erected
and made strait for the passage of the penis in the
womb—secondly, whilst the passage is repleted
with spirit and vital blood, it becomes more strait
for embracing the penis; and as for the conveniency of erection, it is two-fold—First, because if
the neck of the womb was not erected, the yard
would have no convenient passage to the womb :

Secondly it hinders any hurt or damage that might ensue through the violent concussion of the yard, during the time of copulation.

As for the veins that pass through the neck of the womb, their voice is to replenish it with blood and spirit, that still as the moisture consumes by the heat contracted in copulation, it may by these vessels be renewed; but their chief business is to convey nutriment to the womb.

The womb has many properties attributed to it. As first, rentention of the foecundated egg, and this is properly called conception. Secondly, to cherish and nourish it till nature has framed the child, and brought it to perfection, and then it strongly operates in sending forth the birth, when the time of its remaining there is expired, dilating itself in a wonderful manner, and so aptly removed from the senses, that nothing of injury can proceed from thence; retaining to itself a power and strength to operate and cast forth the birth, unless by accident it be rendered deficient; and then to strengthen and enable it, remedies must be applied by skilful hands, directions for the applying of which shall be given in the second part.

The use of the preparing vessel is this, the arteries convey the blood of the testicles; part whereof is put in nourishment of them, and the production of those little bladders (in all things resembling eggs) through which the vasa preparentia runs, and are obliterated in them; and as for the veins their office is to bring back what blood remains from the use aforesaid.

The vessels of this kind are much shorter in women than in men, by reason of their nearness to the stones, which defects is yet made good by the many intricate windings to which those vessels are subject; for in the middle way they divide themselves, into two branches, though different In magnitude, for one being greater than the other passes to the stones.

The stones in woman are very useful, for where they are defective; generation work is at an end; for although these bladders which are on their outward superfices contain nothing of seed, as the followers of Galen and Hippocrates did'erroniously imagine yet they contain several eggs, generally 20 (in which testicle) one of each being impregnated by the spiritous part of the man's seed in the act of coition, desends through the oviducts in the womb, and from hence in the process of time becomes a living child.

C H A P. XVI.

Of the Organs of Generation of Man.

HAVING given you a description of the organs of generation in woman, with the anetony of the fabric of the womb; I shall now (to compleat the first part of this treatise) describe the orgins of generation in man, and how they are. fitted to the use for which nature designed them.

The instrument of generation in man (commonly called the yard; and in Lattin, penis a pedendo because it hangs without the belly) is an organical part, which consists of skin, tendons, veins, arteries, sinews and great ligaments; and is long and round, and on the upper side flatish, seated under the ossa pubis, and ordained by nature partly by evacuation of urine, and partly for conveying the seed into the matrix; for which end it is full of small pores through which the seed passes into it, through the vesicula seminalis, and also the neck of the ve-

G

sicula urinalis' which pours out the urine when
they make water; besides the common parts as
caticula, the skin and the membrana carnos it hath
these proper internal parts, viz.   The two nervous
bodies, the septum, the urethera, the glans, four
muscles, and the vessels.   The nervous bodies
(so called) are surrouuded with a thick white previous membrane, but their inmost substance is spungy, consisting chiefley of veins, arteries and nervous fibres intervoven together like a net; and
when the nerves are filed with animal spirits. and
the arteries with hot and spiritous blood, then
the penis is distended and becomes erect; but
when the influx of dead spirits ceases, then the
blood and remaining spirits limber and grow flag-
gy; below these nervous bodies is the uthera,
and whenever the nervous bodies swell, it swells
also.   The muscles of the penis are four, two
shorter rising from the coxendix, and serving its
erection, and for that reason are called erectors;
two large proceeding from the spinter of the anu s
and serve to dilate the uretra ejaculation of seed;
and are called dilatantes, or winding. ' At the
end of the penis is the glands covered with a very
thin membrane; by means of which and its nerv-
ous.substance, it becomes more exqusitely sensible,
and is the principal seat of pleasure in copulation.
The utmost covering of the glans is called proepu-
tium a perputondo from being cut off, being that
which the jews cut off in circumsision, and it is tied
by the lower part of it to the glands of the foetus,
The penis is also stocked with veins, arteries and
nerves,

The testiculi or stones (so called) because testi-
fying one to be a man; elaborate the blood brought
to them by the spermatic arteries into seed.   They

have coats of two sorts, propper and common; 'the common are two' and invest both the testes. The outermost of the common coats consists of the caticula, or true skin ; and is called the scrotum, hanging out of the abdomen like a purse, the inermost is the membran, carnosa; the proper coats' are also two, the outer called eliotrodes or virginals ; the inner albugidia, into the outer is inserted the cremaster : the upper parts of the testes is fixed ; epidimydes, or pastata, from whence arise the vassa differentia, or ejaculatory which when they come near the neck of the bladder, deposit the seed into the vesicule feminiales, these vesicule feminiales, are two, each like a bunch of grapes, and emit the seed into the urethera, in the act of copulation.

Near them are the prostrate, about the bigness of a walnut and join' to the neck of the bladder. Authors cannot agree about the use of them ; but most are of opinion, that they afford an oily sloppy and fat humour to besmere the urethera, whereby to defend the same from the acrimony of the seed and urine. But the vessels which convey the blood to the testes out of which the seed is made arartriae spermaticae, and are also two. The veins which carry out the remaining blood are two, and have the name of venae spermatcae.

CHAP. XVII.

A Word of Advice to both Sexes ; Being several Directions respecting Copulation.

SINCE nature has implanted in every creature a mutual desire of copulation, for the encrease and propagation of its kind ; and more especially in man, the lord of the creation, and master-piece of nature ; that so noble a piece of divine workmanship might not perish, something ought to be said concerning that, it being the foundation of all that we have been hitherto treating of; since without copulation there can be no generation. Seeing therefore it depends so much upon it, I thought it necessary, before I conclude the first part, to give such directions to both sexes, for the performing of that act, as may appear efficacious to the end for which nature designed it. But it will be done with that caution, as not to offend the chastest ear, nor put the fair sex to the trouble of a blush in reading it. Therefore, when a married couple, from a desire of having children, are about to make use of those means that nature ordained to that purpose, it would be very proper to cherish the body with generous restoratives, so that it may be brisk and vigorous : and if their imaginations were charmed with sweet and melodious airs, and cares and thoughts of business drowned in glass of racy wine, that their spirits may be raised to the highest pitch of ardor and joy, it would not be amiss. For any thing of sadness, trouble and sorrow, are enemies to delights of Venus. And if at such times of coition, there should be conception, it would have a malevolent effect upon children. But though generous restoratives may be used for invigorating nature, yet all excess is carefully to be avoided, for it will allay the briskness of the spirits, and render them dull and languid, and also hinders digestion, and so must needs be an enemy to copulation. For if food moderately taken that is well digested, creates good spirits, and enables a man with vigour and activity to perform the dictates of nature. It is also highly necessary, that, in their natural embraces, they meet each other with an equal ardor. For if the spirits flag on each other, they will fall short of what nature requires : and women either miss of conception, or else the children prove weak in their bodies, or defective in their understanding : and therefore I do advise them before they begin their conjugal embraces, to invigorate their mutual desires, and make their flames burn with a fierce ardor, by those endearing ways, that love can better teach than I can write.

When they have done what nature requires, a man must have a care he does not part too soon, from the embraces of his wife, lest some sudden interposing cold should strike into the womb, and occasion miscarriage, and thereby deprive them of the fruit of their labour.

And when after some small convenient time the man hath withdrawn himself, let the woman gently betake herself to rest with all imaginable serenity and composure of mind, from all anxious and disturbing thoughts, or any other kind of pertubation : And let her, as much as she can, forbear turning herself from that side on which she first reposed ; and by all means let her avoid coughing or sneezing, which, by its violent concussion of the body, is a great enemy to conception, if it happen soon after the act of coition. -

The End of the First Book.

A
Private Looking-Glass

PART SECOND.

*Treating of Several Maladies incident to the womb;
with proper remedies for the cure of each.*

CHAP. I.

Of the Womb in general.

ALTHOUGH in the First Part I have spoken
something of the fabric of the womb, yet
being in the Second Part to treat more particularly
hereof, and of the various distempers and maladies,
it is subject to ; I shall not think it tautology, to
give you, by way of instruction, a general description both of its situation and parts, but rather
think this Second Part would be imperfect without
it, can by no means be omitted, especially since in
it I am to speak of the menstruous blood.

First—Touching the Womb : Of the Grecian it
is called Metra, the mother ; Adelphos saith Pris-
cian, because it makes us all brothers.

It is placed in hypogastrum, or lower part of
the body, in the cavity called pelvis, having the
strait gut on one side, to keep it from the other side
of the back bone, and the bladder on the other side
to defend it from blows. The form or figure of it
is like a virile member, only this excepted ; the
manhood is outward, and womanhood within.

It is divided into the neck and the body : The

traversely placed, called hymen, or engion; near unto the neck there is a prominant pinnacle, which is called of Montanus, the door of the womb, because it preserveth the matrix from the cold and dust. Of the Grecians it is called clytoris, of the Latins perputium muliebre, because the Jewish women did abuse those parts to their own mutual lusts, as St. Paul speaks, Rom. i. 26.

The body of the womb is that wherein the child is conceived. And this is not altogether round, but dilates itself into two angles; the outward part of it is nervous and full of sinews, which are the cause of its motion, but inwardly it is fleshy. It is fabulously reported, that in the cavity of the womb there are seven divided cells, or receptacles for human seed. But those that have seen anatomies, do know there are but two; and likewise, that these two are not divided by a partition, but only by a line, running through the midst of it. In the right side of the cavity, by reason of the left side, by the coldness of the spleen females are begotten.

And this do most of our moderns hold for an infallible truth, yet Hippocrates holds it but in the general: For in whom, saith. he, the spermatic vessels on the right side come from the reins, and the spermatic vessels on the left side from the hollow veins, in them males are conceived in the left side, and the females in the right. Well, therefore, may I conclude with the saying of Epidocles —Such sometimes is the power of the seed, that a male may be conceived in the left side, as well as in the right. In the bottom of the cavity there are little holes called the cotilendons, which are the end of certain veins and arteries, serving in breeding women to convey substance to the child which is received by the umbilical veins; and, others to carry the courses into the matrix.

Now touching the menstruels—they are defined
to be a monthly flux of excrementious and unpro-
fitable blood.

In which we are to note, that the matter flowing
forth is excrementitious ; which is to be understood
of the superplus or redundance of it, for it is an
excrement in quality, its quantity being pure and
incorrupt, like unto the blood in the veins.

And that the menstruous blood is pure and subtile of itself, all in one quality with that in the veins,
is proved two ways : First from the final cause of
the blood, which is the propagation and conserva-
tion of mankind; that man might be conceived,
and being begotten, he might be comforted and
preserved both in the womb and out of the womb.
And all will grant it for a truth, that a child while
it is in the matrix, nourished with the blood ; and
it is true, that being out of the womb it is still
nourished with the same, for the milk is nothing
but the menstruous blood made white in the
breast; and I am sure women's milk is not thought
to be venomous, but of a putritive quality, answer-
able to the tender nature of the infant. Secondly—
It is proved to be true from the generation of it,
it being the superfluity of the last aliament of the
fleshy part.

It may be objected—If the body be not of a hurtful quality, how can it cause such venomous effects?
As if the same fall upon trees and herbs, it maketh
the one barren, and mortifieth the other. Averves
writes ; That if a man accompany with any menstrous women, if she conceive she shall bring forth
a leper. I answer—This mallgnity is contracted
in the womb ; for that wanting native heart to digest thi superfluity, sends it to the matrix, where
seatling itself until the mouth of the womb be di-

lated, it becomes corrupt and venemous, which may easily be, considering the heat and moisture of the place. This blood, therefore, being out of its vessels, it offends in quality. In this sense let us understand Pliny, Cornelius Florns, and the rest of that torrent. But if frigidity be the cause why women cannot digest all their last nourishments, and consequently that they have these purgations, it remains to give a reason why they are of so cold a constitution more than a man which is this.

The natural end of man and woman's being is to propagate; and this injunction was imposed upon them by God at their first creation, and again after the deluge. Now in the act of conception there must be an agent and patient, for if they be both every way of one constitution, they cannot propagate; man therefore, is hot and dry, woman cold and moist; he is the agent, she the patient, or weaker vessel, that she should be subject to the office of the man. It is necessary the woman should be of a cold constitution, because in her is required a redundancy of nature for the infant depending on her; for otherwise, if there were not a superplus of nourishment for the child, more than is convenient for the mother, then would the infant detract and weaken the principal parts of the mother, and like unto the viper, the generation of the infant, would be the destruction of the parent.

The monthly purgations continue from the fifteenth year to the forty-sixth or fiftieth. Yet often there happen a suppression, which is either natural or morbifical, they are naturally supprest in breeding women, and such as are sick. The morbifical suppression falls into our method to be spoken of.

GHAP. II.

Of the Retention of the Courses.

THE suppression of the terms is an intercep-
tion of that customary evacuation of blood,
which, every month, should come from the matrix, proceed from the instrument or matter vitiated, the part affected is the womb, and that of
itself or by consent.

CAUSE.]—The cause of this suppression is either external or internal. The external cause
may be heat or dryness of the air, immoderate
watching, great labour, vehement motion, &c.
whereby the matter is confused, and the body so
exhausted, that there is not a superplus remaining
to be expelled as is recorded of the Amazons,
who being active and always in motion, had their
fluxations very little. or not at all. Or, it may
be caused by cold. which is most frequent, making
the blood vicious and gross, condensing and binding up the passages that it cannot flow forth.

The internal cause is either instrumental or
material —in the womb or in the blood.

In the womb it may be divers ways ; by a post-
humes, humours, ulcers, by the narrowness of the
veins and passages, or. by the omentum or kell in
fat bodies. pressing the neck of the matrix ; but
then they must have hernia zirthilis ; for in mankind the kell reacheth not so low. By over-much
cold or heat. the one vitiating the action, and the
other consuming the matter by an evil composition of the uterine parts, by the neck of the womb
being turned aside, and sometimes. though rarely,
by a membrane or excrescence of the flesh growing about the mouth or neck of the womb.   The

blood may be in fault two ways, in quaniity or quality. In quantity, when it is so consumed that there
is not a superplus left, as in virgoes or virile women, who, thro' their heat and strength of nature,
digest and consume all in their last nourishment.

SIGNS.] Signs manifesting the disease, are pains
in the head, neck, back and loins, weariness of the
whole body, but especially of the hips and legs, by
reason of a confinity which the matrix hath with
these parts,trembling of the heart ; particular signs
are these—if the suppression proceed from cold,
she is heavy, sluggish, of a pale colour, and has a
slow pulse ; Venus's combats are neglected, the
urine crudle, waterish, and much in quantity, the
excrements of the guts usually are retained. If of
that, the signs are contrary to those now recited.
If the retention be natural, and come of conception,
this may be known by drinking of hydromel, that
is, water and honey, after supper, going to bed, and
by the effect which it worketh ; for, after taking it,
she feels a beating pain upon the navel, and lower
part of the belly, it is a sign she hath conceived,
and that the suppression is natural ; if not, then it is
vicious, and ought medicinally to be taken away.

PROGNOSTICS.]—With the evil quality of the
womb the whole body stands charged, but especially the heart, the liver, and the brain : and betwixt
the womb and these three principal parts, there is a
singular concert. First,the womb communicates to
the heart, by the mediation of those arteries which
come from aorta. Hence, the terms being supprest,
will ensue faintings,swoonings,intermission of pulse
cessation of breath. Secondly, it communicates to
to the liver, by the veins derived from the hollow
vein. Then will follow obstructions, cahexies,
jaundies, dropsies, hardness of spleen, Thirdly it

it communicats to the brain, by the nervse & membrane of the back ; hence will arrise epilepsies,
frenzies melancholy, passion, pain in the after-part
of the head, fearfulness, inability of speaking.
Well, therefore, may I conclude with Hipocrates—
If the months be suppress, many dangerous diseases will follow.

CURE.]—In the cure of this, and of all other following effects, I will observe this order. The cure
must be taken from chirugical, pharmacutical and
diuretical means. This suppression is a phletoric
effect, and must be taken away by evacuation. And
therefore we will first begin with phlebotomy. In
the midst of the menstrual period, open the liver
vein ; and, for the reversion of the humour, two
days before the wonted evacuation, open the saphena on both feet ; if the repletion be not great, apply cupping-glasses to the legs and thighs, although
there be no hope to remove the suppression.

After the humour hath been purged, proceed to
make proper and forcible remedies. Take of trochisk of myrh one dram and a half, parsley-seed,
castor rhinds, or cassia, of each one scruple, and of
the extract of mugwort one scruple and an half,
musk ten grains, with the jsuie of smallage, make
twelve pills, take six every morning, or after supper, going to bed.

If the retention comes from repletion or fulness,
let the air be hot and dry, use moderate exercise
before meals, and your meat and drink attenuating ;
seethe, with your meat, garden savory, thyme, ori-
gane, and cyche peason ; if of emptiness, or defect
of matter, let the air be moist and moderate hot,
shun exercise and watchings, let your meat be nourishing and of a light digestion, as rare eggs, lamb,
chickens, almonds, zilik, and the like.

CHAP. III.

Of the Overflowing of the Courses.

THE learned say, by comparing of contraries truth is made manifest. Having, therefore, spoken of the suppression of terms, order requires, now that I should insist on the overflowing of them, an effect no less dangerous than the former and this immoderate flux if the month is defined to be a sanguinous excrement proceeding from the womb, exceeding in both qnantity and time : First it is said to be sanguinous, the matter of the flux being only blood wherein it differs from that which is commonly called the false courses or whites, of which I shall speek hereafter. Secondly, it is said to proceed from the womb, for there are two ways by which the blood flows forth, the one way is by the internal veins in the body of the womb, and this is properly called the monthly flux. The other is by those veins which are terminated in the neck of the womb. Lastly, it is said to exceed both in quantity and time. In quantity, saith Hipocrates, when they flow about eighteen ounces ; in time, when they flow above three days; but we take this for a certain character of their inordinate flowing, when the faculties of the body thereby are weakened ; in bodies abounding with gross humours, this immoderate flux sometimes unburthens nature of her load, and ought not be stayed without the consent of a physician.

'CAUSE.]—The cause of this affair is internal or external ; the internal cause is threefold, in the matter, instrument, or faculty : The matter, which is in the blood, may be vicious two ways—First, by the heat of constitution, climate or season heating the blood, whereby the passages are dilated, and

H..

the faculty weakened, that it cannot contain the blood. Secondly, by falls, blows, violent motion, breaking of the veins, &c.

The external cause may be calidity of the air, lifting, carrying of heavy burdens, unnatural child-birth, &c.

SIGNS.] – In this inordinate flux, the appetite is decayed, the conception deprived, and all the actions weakened, the feet are swelled, the colour of the face is chang'd, and a general feebleness possesseth the whole body. If the flux comes by the breaking of a vein, the body is sometimes cold, the blood flows forth on heaps, and that suddenly, with great pains. If it comes through heat, the orifice of the vein being dilated, then there is little or no pain ; yet the blood flows laster than it doth in an erosion, and not so fast as it doth in a rupture. If by erosion, or sharpness of blood, she feels a great heat scalding the passage, it differs from the other two, in that it flows not so suddenly, nor so copiously as they do : If by-weakness of the womb, she abhorreth the use of Venus. Lastly, if it proceed' from an evil quality of the blood, drop some of it on a cloth, and when it is dry, you may judge of the quality of the colour. If it be choleric, it will be yellow ; if melancholy, black ; if plegmatic, waterish and whitish.

PROGNOSTICS.]—If with the flux be joined a convulsion, it is dangerous, because it intimates the more noble parts are vitiated, and a convulsion caused by emptiness is deadly ; If it continues long, it will be cured with great difficulty, for it was one of the miracles that our Saviour Chrsit wrought; to cure this disease, when it had contined twelve years. To conclude, If the flux be inordinate, many diseases will ensue, and, without remedy, the blood, together with the native heat, being consumed, either cachectical, hydropical, or pareletical diseases will follow.

Cure.]—The cure consisteth in three particulars: First, in repelling and carrying away the blood.—Secondly, in correcting and taking away the fluxability of the matter. Thirdly, in corroborating the veins and faculties: For the first, to cause a regression of the blood, open a vein in the arm, and draw out so much blood as the strength of the patient will permit; and that not together, but at several times for thereby the spirits are less weakened, and the refraction so much the greater.

Apply cupping-glasses to the breasts, and also the liver, that the reversion may be in the fountain.

To correct the fluxability of the matter, cathartical means, moderated with the astrictories, may be used.

If it be caused by erosion, or sharpness of blood, consider whether the orosion be by salt phlegm, or adust choler; it with salt phlegm, prepare with syrup of violets, wormwood, roses, citron-peel, succory, &c. Then take this purgation following: Mirobulana, chebol half an ounce, trochilks of agaric one dram, with plaintain water, make a decoction, add thereunto fir, roseat, lax three ounces, and make a potion.

If by adust choler, prepare the body with syrup of roses, myrtles, sorrel, purslain, mix with water of plaintain, knot-grass and endive—then purge with this potion: Take rhind of mirobulana, rhubarb, of each one dram, cinnamon fiteen grains, infuse them one night in endive water; and to the straining pulp of a tamarind, cassia, of each half an ounce, syrup of roses an ounce, make a potion:—
If the blood be waterish or unconcoct, as it is in

the hydropical bodies, and flow forth by reason of the tenuity or thinness to draw off the water, it will be profitable to purge with agaric elaterium, coloquintida : Sweating is proper in this case, for thereby the matter offending is taken away, and the motion of the blood carried to the outward parts. To procure sweat, use carduus water, with mythridate, or the decoction of sarsaparilla: The gum of guaiacum also greatly provokes sweat; pills of sarsaparilla, taken every night going to bed, are worthily commended. If the blood flows forth through the opening or breaking of a vein, without any evil quality of itself, then ought only corroboratives to be applied, which is the last thing to be done in this inordinate flux.

The air must be cold and dry ; all motion of the body is forbidden ; let her meat be pheasant, partridge, mountain-birds, coneys, calves' feet, &c.—And let her beer be mixt with the juice of pomegranates and quinces.

CHAP. IV.

Of the Weeping of the Womb.

THE weeping of the womb is a flux of blood, unnatural, coming from thence in drops, after the manner of tears, causing violent pains in the same, keeping neither period nor time. By some it is referred unto the immoderate evacuation of the course, yet they are distinguished in the quantity and manner of overflowing. in that they flow copiously and free in this continually, though by little and little, and that with great pain and difficulty, wherefore, it is likened unto the stranguary.

The cause is in the faculty, instrument, or matter. In the faculty; by being enfeebled, that it cannot expel the blood, and the blood resting there, makes the part of the womb grow hard, and stretcheth the vessels from whence preceedeth the pain of the womb : In the instrument, by the narrowness of the passages. Lastly, it may be the matter of the blood, which may offend in too great a quantity, or in an evil quality, it being gross and thick, that it cannot flow forth as it ought to do, but by drops. The signs will best appear by the relation of the patient : Hereupon will issue pains in the head, stomach, and back, with inflammations in the head, stomach, and back ; with inflammation, suffocations and excoriations of the matrix : If the strength of the patient will permit first open a vein in the arm, rub the upper parts, and let her arm be corded, that the force of the blood may be carried backwards ; then apply such things as may laxate and mollify the strengthening the womb, and assuage the sharpness of the blood, as cataplasms made of brand; lintseed, fenugreek, meliot, mallows, mercury and artiplex : If the blood be vicious and gross, add thereto mugwort, calamint, dictam and betony ; and let her take of Venice treacle the quantity of a nutmeg, the syrup of mugwort every morning, make injections of the decoctions of mallows, mercury, lintseed, grounsel, mugwort, fenugreek, with oil of sweet almonds.

Sometimes it is oaused by wind, and then phlebotome is to be omitted, and in the stead thereof take syrup of feferfew an ounce, honey; roses, syrup of roses, syrup of flæchus, of each half an oz. Water of calamint, mugwort, betony, hysop, of each an oz, make a julep ; if the pain continues, take this purgation—take spechieiæ one diam diacatholicon half an oz, syrup of roses, laxaivets

H 2
H 2

one ounce, with the decoction of mugwort, and the four cordial flowers, make a potion. If it comes through the weakness of the faculty, let that be corroborated—If through the grossness and sharpness of the blood, let the quality of it be altered, as I have shewn in the foregoing chapter.— Lastly, If the excrements of the guts be retained, provoke them by glyster of the decoction of camomile, betony, feverfew, mallows, lintseed, juniper-berries, common seed, anniseed, meliote, adding thereto diacatholicon half an ounce, salt nitre a dram and a half. The patient must abstain from salt, sharp and windy meat.

CHAP. V.

The false Courses, or Whites.

FROM the womb proceeds not only menstruous blood, but, accidentally, many other excrements, which, by the ancients, are comprehended under the title of robus, gunakois, which is a distillation of a variety of corrupt humours through the womb, flowing from the whole body, or part of the same, keeping neither course nor colour, but varying in both.

Course.]—The cause is either promiscuously in the whole body, by a cacochymia, or weakness of the same, or in some of the parts, as in the liver, which by the inability of the sanguifacative faculty, causeth a generation of corrupt blood ; and the matter is reddish, sometimes the gall being sluggish in its office, not drawing away those choleric superfluities engendered in the liver; and the matter is yellowish sometimes in the spleen, not descending and cleansing the blood of the dregs of excrementious parts. And then, the matter flow-

ing forth is blackish : It may also come from the
cattarahs in the head, or from any other putrified
or corrupted member ; but if the matter of the flux
be white, the cause is either in the stomach or
reins. In the stomach, by a phlegmatical and crude
matter there contracted and variated, thro' grief,
melancholy, and other distempers ; for, otherwise,
if the matter were only pernical, crude, phlegm,
and no ways corrupt, being taken into the liver, it
might be converted into blood ; for, phlegm in the
ventricle is called nourishments half digested ; but
being corrupt, though sent into the liver, yet it
cannot be turned into nutriment ; for, the second
decoction cannot correct that which the first hath
corrupted ; and therefore the liver sends it to the
womb, which can neither digest nor repel it, and
so it is voided out with the same colour it had in
the ventricle.—The cause also may be in the reins
being over-heated, whereby the spermatical matter, by reason of its thinness flows forth. The
external causes may be moistness of the air, eating of corrupt meats, anger, grief, slothfulness,
immoderate sleeping, costiveness in the body.

The signs are, exturbation of the body, shortness
and stinking of the breath, loathing of meat, pain
in the head, swelling in the eyes and feet, melan-
cholly ; humidity flows from the womb of divers
colours, as red, black, green, yellow and white. It
differs from the flowing and overflowing of the
courses, in that it keeps no certain period, and is of
many colours, all which do generate from blood.

PROGNOSTICS.]—If the flux be phlegmatical, it
will continue long, and be difficult to cure ; yet, if
mitting, for diarhæ happeneth, diverts the humour,
it cures the disease. If it be choleric, it is not so
permanent, yet more perilous, for it will cause a

cliff in the neck of the womb, and sometimes make
an excoriation of the matrix; in melancholic it
must be dangerous contamacious ; yet the flux of
the hemerhoids administers cure.

If the matter flowing forth be reddish, open a
vein in the arm ; if not, apply ligatures to the arms
and shoulders : Galen glories of himself, how he
cured the wife of Brutus laboring of this disease,
by rubbing the upper part with crud honey.

If it is caused by distillation from the brain take
syrup of betony, stochas and marjoram, purge with
pilloch, fine quibus de agarico ; make nasalia of
of the juice of sage, hyssop betony, nigella, with
one drop of the oil of elect, dianth, aromat, rosat,
diambræ, diomeseth, dulcis, of each on dram ; nutmeg, half a dram ; with sugar and betony water,
make lozenges, to be taken every morning and
evening. Huri Alexandrina half a dram, at night
going to bed.   If these things help not, use the
suffumigation and plaister, as they are prescribed.

If it proceeds from crudities in the stomach, or
from a cold distempered liver, take every morning
of the decoction of lignum sanctum ; purge with
pill de agarico, de hermodact, de hiera, diacolin-
thid, fœtid, agrigatio ; take elect. aromat, roses,
two drams ; citron pill dried, nutmeg, long pepper, of each one scruple, with mint water, and
make lozenges of it. Take of them before meals ;
if the frigidity of the liver there be joined a repletion of the stomach, purging by vomit is commen-
dable ; for which take three drams of the electuary diasara Galen allows of diuretical means as ab-
sum, ptroso linan.

If the matter of the flux be choleric, prepare the
humour with syrup of roses, violets, endive, succory ; purge with mirobolans, manna, rhubarb, cassia.

Take of rhubarb two drams, anniseed one dram, cinnamon a scruple and an half; infuse them in six ounces prune broth; add too the straining of manna an ounce, and take in the morning according to art. Take spicerum, diatonianton, diacorant, prig diarthod; abbaris, diacydomes, of each one dram, sugar four ounces, with plaintain water, make lozenges, If the clyster of the gall be sluggish, and do not stir up the faculty of the gut, give glysters, with the decoction of four molifying herbs, with honey of roses and aloes.

If the flux be melancholous, prepare with syrup of maiden hair, epithymium, polipedy, borrage buglos, fumitary, harts tongue, and syrupus bisatius, which must be made without vinegar, otherwise it will rather animate the disease than nature; for melancholy, by the use of vinegar, is encreased, and both by Hippocrates, Sylvius, and Avenzoar, it is disallowed of as an enemy to the womb, and therefore not to be used inwardly in all uterine diseases.

Lastly—Let the womb be cleansed from the corrupt matter, and then corroborated; for the purifying thereof make injections of the decoction of betony, feverfew, spikenard bistrop, mercury, sage, adding thereto sugar, oil of sweet almonds, of each two ounces; pessaries also may be made of silk, cotton, modified in the juice of the aforementioned herbs.

CHAP. VI.

Of the Suffocation of the Mother.

THE effect (which if simply considered) is none but the cause of an effect, is called in English the suffocation of the mother; not because

the womb is strangled, but for that it causeth the
womb to be choaked.   It is a retraction of the
womb towards the: midriff and stomach, which
presseth and crusheth up the same, that the instrumental cause of respiration, the midriff is suffocated—and consenting with the brain, causing
the animating faculty, the efficient cause of respiration, also to be intercepted, where the body being refrigerated and the action depraved, she falls
to the ground as one being dead.

In these hysterical passions some continue longer
some shorter: Rabbi Moses writes of some who
lay in the paroxysy of the fit for two days.   Ru-
fus makes mention of one who continued in the
same passion three days and three nights, and at
the three days end she revived.   That we may
learn by other men's harms to beware, I will tell
you an example, Parœus writeth of a woman in
Spain who suddenly fell into an uterine suffocation
and appeared to men's judgment as dead ; her
friends wondering at this her sudden change, for
their better satisfaction sent for a surgeon to have
her dissected, who beginning to make an incision,
the woman began to move, and with great clamour
returned to herself again, to the horror and ad-
miration of all the spectators.

That you may distinguish the living from the
dead, the ancients prescribe three experiments :
The first is to lay a light feather to the mouth, and
by its motion you may judge whether the patient
be living or dead.   The second is—to place a glass
of water on the breast, and if you perceive it to
move, it betokeneth life.   The third is—to hold a
pure looking-glass to the mouth and nose, and if
the glass appears thick with a little dew upon it,
it betokeneth life.   And these three experiments

are good, yet with this caution, that you ought not to depend on them too much, for though the feather and the water do not move, and the glass continue pure and clear, yet it is not a necessary consequence that she is destitute of life ; for the motion of the lungs, by which the respiration is made, may be taken away that she cannot breathe, yet the internal transpiration of the heat may re-main, which is not manifest by the motion of the breast or lungs, but lies occult in the heart and in-ward arteries ; examples thereof we have in the fly and swallow, which in the cold of winter seem dead, and breath not at all ; yet they live by the transpiration of that heat which is reserved in the heart and inward arteries ; therefore when the summer approacheth, the internal heat being re-vocated to the inward parts, they are then again revived out of their sleepy ecstacy.

Those women therefore that seem to die sud-den, and upon no evident cause, let them not be committed to the earth unto the end of three days, lest the living be buried for the dead.

Cause.]—The part affected in the womb, of which there are a twofold motion, natural and symptomatical. The natural motion is, when the womb attracteth the human seed, or excludeth the infant or secundine. The symptomatical motion of which we are to speak, is a convulsive drawing of the womb.

Signs.]—At the approaching of the suffocation, there is a paleness of the face, weakness of the legs, shortness of breath, frigidity of the whole body, with a working up into the throat, and then she falls down at once void both of sense and motion ; the mouth of the womb is closed up, and being touched with the finger it feels hard, the paroxism of the fit one past, she openeth her eyes, and feeling her stomach opprest, she offers to vomit.

'Prognostics'.]—If the disease hath its being from the corruption of the seed, it foretels more danger than if it proceeded from the suppression of the courses, because the seed is concocted and of a purer quality than the menstruous blood; and the more pure being corrupted, becomes the more foul and filthy, as appears in eggs the purest nourishment which vitiated, will yield the noisomest favour. If it be accompanied with a syncope, it shews nature is but weak, and that the spirits are almost exhausted; but 'if sneezing follows, it shews the heat that was almost extinct, doth now begin to return, and nature will subdue the disease.

Cure.]—In the cure of this effect, two things must be observed : First, That during the time of the paroxism, nature be provoked to expel those malignant vapours which bind up the senses, that she may be recalled out of the sleepy exstacy. Secondly, That in the intermission of the fit, proper medicines be applied to take away the cause.

To stir up nature, fasten cupping-glasses to the hips and navel, applying ligatures unto the thighs ; rub the extreme parts with salt, vinegar, and mustard; cause loud clamours and thunderings in the ears. Apply to the nose assafœtida castor, and sagapanenm steeped in vinegar, provoke her to sneeze by blowing up into her nostrils the powder of castor, white pepper, pellitory of Spain, and hellebore. Hold under her nose patridge feathers, hair and old shoes burnt, and all other stinking things, for evil odours are an enemy to nature ; hence the animal spirits do so contest and strive against them that the natural heat is thereby restored. The brain is so opprest sometimes, that we are compelled to burn the outward skin of the head with hot oil, or with a hot iron. Sharp clysters and suppositories are available. Take of sage, calamint, harehound, feverfew, marjoram, betyon, hyssop, of each one handful; anniseed half an ounce; coloquotinda, white hellebore, sal gem. of each two drams; boil these in two pounds of water to the half; add to the straining oil of castor two ounces; hiera picra two drams, and make a glyster of it.

If it be caused by the retention and corruption of the seed, at the instant of the paroxism, let the midwife take oil of lilies, margoram and bays, dissolving in the same two grains of civet; add as much musk; let her dip her finger therein, and put into the neck of the womb, tickling and rubbing the same.

The fit being over, proceed to the curing of the cause. If from the retention of the seed, a good husband will administer a cure, but those who cannot honestly purchase that cure, must use such things as will dry up and diminish the seed; as dicuminua, diacalaminthes, &c. Amongst banonics, the seed of augus castus is well esteemed of, whether taken inwardly applied outwardly, or receive a suffumigation. It was held in great honor amongst the Athenians, for by it they did remain as pure vessels, and preserved their chastity by only strowing it on the bed whereon they lay, and hence the name of augus castus given it, as denoting its effects. Make an issue in the inside of each leg, an hand breadth below the knee. Make trochisks of agric two scruples, wild carrot-seed, lign aloes, of each half a scruple; washed turpentine, three drams, with conserve of anthos make a bolus; castor is of excellent use in this case, eight

drams of it taken in white wine, or you may make
pills of it with mithridite, and take them going to
bed. Take of the white briony root dried, and after
the manner of carrots, one ounce; put into a
draught of wine, placing it by the fire, and when
it is warm drink it; take myrrh, castor, asofœtida,
of each one scruple; saffron and rue seed, of each
four grains; make eight pills, and take two every
night going to bed.

Galen, by his own example, commends unto us
agaric pulverized, of which he frequently gave one
scruple in white wine : lay to the navel at bed time
a head of garlic bruised, fastening it with a swith-
ing-band ; make a girdle of galbacum for the waist,
and also a plaister for the belly, placing in one part
of it civet and musk, which must be laid upon the
navel.   Take pulveris benedict, trochisk of agaric,
of each two drams mithridite a sufficient quantity,
and so make two passeries, and it will purge the
matrix of wind and phlegm, foment the natural
part with salad oil, in which has been boiled rue,
feverfew and camomile.

CHAP. VII.

Of descending or falling of the Mother.

THE falling down of the womb is relaxation of
the ligatures, whereby the matrix is carried
backward, and in some hangs out in the bigness
of an egg.   Of these there are two kinds, distinguished by a descending and precipitation.   The
descending of the womb is, when it sinks down
to the entrance of the privities, and appears
to the eye either not at all or very little.   The
precipitation is, when the womb, like a purse
is turned inside outward, and hangs betwixt the

thighs in the bigness of a cupping-glass.

Cause.]—the cause is external or internal : The external cause is difficult child-birth, violent pulling away the secundine, rashness and inexperience in drawing away the child, violent coughing, sneezing, falls, blows, and carrying heavy burthens.— The internal cause, in general, is overmuch humidity flowing into these parts, hindering the operation of the womb, whereby the ligaments by which the womb is supported is relaxed.

The cause, in particular, is referred to be in the retention of the seed, or in the suppression of the monthly courses.

Signs.]—The a—e, gut and bladder oftentimes are so crushed that the passage of both excrements are hindered ; if the urine flows forth white and thick, and the midriff is molested, the lions are grieved, the privities pained, and the womb sinks down to the private parts, or else comes clean out.

Prognostics.]—This grief possessing an old woman is cured with great difficulty, because it weakens the faculty of the womb, and therefore though it be reduced into its proper place, yet upon very little illness or indisposition it is subject to return ; and so it also is with the younger sort, if the disease be inveterate. If it be caused by a putrefaction in the nerves it is incurable.

Cure.]—The womb being naturally placed between the strait. gut and the bladder, and now fallen down, ought to be put up again, until the faculty both of the gut and bladder be stirred up ; nature being unloaded of her burden, let the woman be laid on her back in such sort, that her legs may be higher than her head ; let her feet be drawn up to her hinder parts, with her knees spread abroad ; then molify the swelling with oil

of lillies and sweet almonds, or with the decoction
of mallows, beets, fenugrek, and lintseed : When
the inaflmation is dissipated, let the midwife anoint
her hand with oil of mastick, and reduce the womb
into its place.

CHAP. VIII.
Of the Inflamation of the Womb.

THE phlegmon, or inflammation of the matrix,
is an humour possessing the whole womb,
acompanied with unnatural heat, by obstruction
and gathering together of corrupt blood

Cause.] The cause of this effect is suppression of
the menses, repletion of the whole body, immoderate
use of Venus, often handling the genitals, difficult
child-birth, vehement agitation of the body, falls,
blows ; to which also may be added, the use of
sharp pessaries, whereby not seldom the womb is inflamed ; cupping-glasses also fastened to the pubis
and hypogastrium, draw the humours to the womb.

Signs.] The signs are anguish, humours, pain in
the head and stomach, vomiting, coldness of the
knees, convulsions of the neck, doating, trembling
of the heart ; often there is a straitness of breath, by
reason of the heat which is communicated to the
midriff, the breasts sympathizing with the womb,
pained and swelled, Further, if the fore-part of the
matrix be inflamed, the privities are grieved, the
urine is supprest, or flows forth with difficulty. If
the after-part, the loins and back suffer, the excrements are retained ; if the right side, the right hip
suffers, the right leg is heavy, slow to motion, inso-
much that sometimes she seems to halt. And so, if
the left side of the womb be inflamed, the left hip
is pained, and the left leg is weaker than the right.

If the neck of the womb be refreshed, the midwife putting up her fiager, shall feel the mouth of
it retracted, and closed up with hardness about it.

Prognostics.]—All· inflammations of the womb
are dangerous, if not deadly ; and especially if the
total substance of the matrix be inflamed ; yet, they
are perilous if in the neck of the womb. A flux of
the belly foretells health, if it be natural ; for, nature works best by the use of her own instruments.

Cure.]—In the cure, first let humours flowing
to the womb be repelled ; for effecting of which,
after the belly has been loosened by cooling clysters, phlebotomy will be needful ; open, therefore,
a vein in the arm, and (if she be not with child)
the day after, strike saphena on both feet, fasten
ligatures and cupping-glasses to the arm, and rub
the upper part. Purge lightly with cassia, rhubarb, senna, morobolans. Take of senna two
drams, anniseed one scruple mirobolans, half an
ounce, barley-water a sufficient quantity, make a
decoction: dissolve in it syrup of succory, with
rhubarb, two onnces, pulp of cassia half an ounce,
oil of anniseed two drops, and make a potion

The air must be cold, all motion of the body,
especially of the lower parts, is forbidden ; vigi-
lance is commended ; for, by sleep the humours
are carried inward, by which the inflammation is
increased, eat sparingly, let your drink be barley-
water, clarified whey ; and your meat chickens
and chicken-broth, boiled with endive, succory,
sorrel, bugloss and mallows.

CHAP. IX.

Of the Scirrosity or Hardness of the Womb.

OF phlegmon neglected, or not perfectly, is generated a schirrus of the matrix; which is a hard unnatural swelling, insensibly hindering the operations of the womb, and disposing the whole body to slothfulness.

Cause.]—One cause of this disease may be ascribed to want of judgment in the physician, as many empirics, administering to an inflammation of the womb, do overmuch refrigerate and affringe the humour that it can neither pass backward nor forward—hence, the matter being condensed, degenerates into a lapidious hard substance Other causes may be, suppression of the menstruous retention of the lochia, commonly called the after-purgings, eating of corrupt meats, as in the disordinate longing called pica, to which breeding women are so often subject. It may proceed also from obstructions and ulcers in the matrix, or from evil effects of the liver and spleen.

Signs.] If the bottom of the womb be affected, she feels, as it were, a heavy burden, representing a mole, yet differing, in that the breasts are attenuated, and the whole body waxeth less. If the neck of the womb be affected, no outward humours will appear; the mouth of it is retracted, and being touched with the finger, feels hard, nor can she have the company of a man without great pains and prickings.

Prognostics.] A schirrus confirmed is incurable, and will turn into a cancer or incurable dropsy, and ending in a cancer proves deadly, because the native heat in those parts being almost smothered, can hardly again be restored.

Cure.] Where there is a repletion, phlebotomy is adviseable ; wherefore, opening the medina on both arms, and the saphena on both feet, more es. pecially if the menses be suppressed.

The air must be temperate ; gross, vicious and salt meats are forbidden, as pork, bull's beef, fish, old cheese, &c.

CHAP. X.

Of the Dropsy of the Womb.

THE uterine dropsy is an unnatural swelling, elevated by the gathering together of wind or phlegm in the cavity, membranes or substance of the womb, by reason of the debility of the native heat and aliment received, and so it turns into an excrement.

The causes are, over-much cold or moistness of the melt and liver, immoderate drinking eating of crude meats, all which causing a repletion, do suf. focate the natural heat. It may be caused likewise by the overflowing of the courses, or by any other immoderate evacuation. To these may be added, abortives, phlegmons and schirrossities of the womb.

Signs.] The signs of this effect are those, the lower parts of the belly, with the genitals, are puff. ed up and pained, the feet swell, the natural colour of the face decays, the appetite is depraved, and the heaviness of the whole body concurs. If she turns herself in the bed, from one side to the other, a noise like the overflowing of water is heard, Water some-times comes from the matrix. If the swelling be caused by wind, the belly being hot, it sounds like a drum ; the guts rumble, and the wind breaks thro' the neck of the womb with a murmuring

noise ; this effect may be distinguished from a true
conception many ways, as will appear by the chapter of conception.

· Prognostics.]—This effect foretell the sad ruin
of the natural functions, by that singular consent
the womb hath with the liver ; that, therefore, the
chacevy, or general dropsy, will follow.

· Cure.]—In the cure of this disease, imitate the
practice of Hippocrates : First, mitigate the pain
with fomentation of melilote, mercury, mallows,
lintseed, camomile, althea. Then let the womb be
prepared with syrup of hyssop, caliment and mugwort. In diseases which have their rise from
moistness, purge with pills. In effects which are
caused by emptiness, or dryness, purge with a potion.—Fasten a cupping-glass to the belly, with a
great fame, and also the navel, especially if the
swelling be flatulent : Make an issue on the inside
of each leg, a hand-breadth below the knee.

The air must be hot and dry, moderate exercise
is allowed ; much sleep is forbidden ; she may eat
the flesh of patridges, larks, chickens, mountain-
birds, hares, conies, &c. Let her drink be thin wine.

CHAP. XI.

Of Moles and false conceptions, ·

THIS disease is called, by the Greeks, mole, and
the cause of this denomination is taken from
the load or heavy weight of it, it being a mole, or
great lump of hard flesh burdening the womb.

· It is defined to be an inarticulate piece of flesh,
without form, begotten in the matrix, as if it were
a true conception. In which definition we are to
note two things : First, in that a mole is said to be
inarticulate, and without form ; it differs from mon-

sters, which are both formate and articulate. Secondly, it is said to be, as it were, a true conception, which puts a difference between a true conception and a mole, which difference holds good three ways: First, in the genus, in that a mole cannot be said to be an animal. Secondly, in the species, because it hath no human figure, and bears not the character of man. Thirdly, in the individum, for it hath no affinity with the parent, either in the whole body, or any particular of the same.

Cause.] About the cause of this effect, amongst learned authors, I find variety of judgments. Some are of opinion, that if the woman's seed goes into the womb, and not the man's, therefore is the mole produced; others there be that affirm, that it is gendered of the menstruous blood. But if these two were granted, then maids, by having their courses, or thro' nocturnal pollutions might be subject to the same, which never yet any were The true cause of this fleshy mole, proceeds both from the man and from the woman, from corrupt and barren seed in man, and from the menstruous blood in woman, both mixed together in the cavity of the womb, where nature finding herself weak, yet desirous of maintaining the perpetuity of her species, labours to bring forth a vicious conception, rather than none ; and so, instead of a living creature, generates a lump of flesh,

Signs.] The signs of a mole are these: The months are suppressed, the appetite depraved, the breasts swell, the belly is suddenly puffed up, and waxeth hard. Thus far the signs of a breeding woman, and one that beareth a mole, are all one. I will shew how they differ: the first sign of difference is taken from the motion of the mole : it may be felt to move in the womb before the 3d month,

which the infant cannot ; yet the motion cannot be
understood of an intelligent power in the mole, but
the faculty of the womb and the seminal spirits
diffused thro' the substance of the mole, for, it lives
not a live animal, but a vegetative, in manner of a
plant. And secondly, in a mole, the belly is suddenly puffed up ; but, in a true conception, the
belly is first retracted, and then riseth up by degrees. Thirdly, the belly being pressed with the
hand, the mole gives way ; and the hand being taken away, it returns to the place again ; but, a child
in the womb, tho' pressed with the hand, moves not
presently,and being removed, returns slowly, or not
at all. Lastly,the children continue in the womb not
above eleven months ; but a mole continues sometimes four or five years, more or less, according as
it is fastened in the matrix. I have known when a
mole hath fallen away in four or five months.

If it remain until the eleventh month, the legs
wax feeble, and the whole body consumes,only the
swelling of the belly still increases ; which makes
some think they are dropsical, tho' there be little
reason for it. For, in the dropsy, legs swell and
grow big, but in a mole they consume and wither.
Prognostics.]—If at the delivery of a mole the
flux of the blood be great, it shews the more danger, because the parts of the nutrition having been
violated by the flowing back of the superfluous humours, where the natural heat is consumed ; and
then parting with so much of blood, the woman
thereby is weakened in all her faculties, that she
cannot subsist without difficulty.

Cure.]—We are taught in the school of Hippocrates, that phlebotomy causeth abortion : by taking all that nourishment which should preserve
the life of the child. Wherefore, that this vi-

cious conception may be deprived of that vegetive sap by which it lives, open the liver vein and the saphena in both the feet; fasten cupping glasses to the loins and sides of the belly, which done let the uterine parts be first molified, and then the expulsive quality be provoked to the burthen.

To laxate the ligature of the mole, take mallows, with the roots three handfuls; camomile, meliloet, pellitory of the wall, violet leaves, mercury, roots of fennel, parsleys of each two hands fuls; lintseed, fenugreek, each one pound; boil them in water, and let her sit therein up to the navel. At the going out of the bath, annoint the privities and reins with this unguent following: Take oil of camomile, lillies, sweet almonds, each one ounce; fresh butter, labdanum, ammoniac, of each an ounce; with the oil of lintseed make an unguent.

The air must be tolerably hot and dry, and dry diet, such as do molify and attenuate, she may drink white wine.

CHAP. XII.

Of the signs of Conception.

IGNORANCE makes women become murderers of the fruit of their own bodies, many having conceived, and thereupon finding themselves out of order, and not knowing rightly the cause, do either run to the shop of their own conceit, and take what they think fit, or else, as the custom is, they send to the physician for a cure; and he not perceiving the cause of their grief, feeling no certain judgment can be given by the urine, prescribes what he thinks best, perhaps some strong dienertic or cathartic potion, whereby the conception is destroyed. Wherefore Hippocrates says, there a necessity that woman should be instructed in the knowledge of conception. that the parent as well as the child might be saved from danger. I will therefore give some instructions by which every one may know whether she be with child or not. The signs of conception shall be taken from the woman, from the urine, from the infant, and from experience.

Signs taken from the woman are these—The first day after conceptiso she feels a light quivering or chillness running through the whole body—a tickling in the womb, a little pain in the lower part of the belly. Ten or twelve days after, the head is affected with giddiness, the eyes with dimness of sight: then follows red pimples in the face, with a blue circle about the eyes, the breast swell and grow hard, with some pain and prickling in them. the belly soon sinketh, and riseth again by degrees. with a hardness about the navel. The nipples of the breast grow red, the heart beats inordinately. the natural appetite is dejected; yet she has a longing desire after meats; the neck of the womb is retracted, that it can hardly be felt with the finger being put up; and this is an infallible sign. She is suddenly merry and soon melancholy, the monthly courses are stayed without any evident cause; the excrements of the guts are unaccustomedly retarded by the womb pressing the great guts, and her desire to Venus is abated.

. The surest sign is taken from the infant, which begins to move in the womb the third or fourth month; and that not in the manner of a male, from one side to another, rustling like a stone, but so softly, as may be perceived by applying the hand hot upon the belly.

Signs taken from the urine ; The best writers do affirm that the urine of a woman with child is white, and hath little mites like those in the sun-beams, ascending and descending in it, a cloud swimming, aloft in an opal colour, the sediments being divided by shaking the urine appears like carded wool, the middle of her time the urine turneth yellow, next red, and lastly black, with a red cloud. Signs taken from experience—At night going to bed let her drink water and honey afterwards, if she feels a beating pain in her belly and about her navel, she hath conceived. Or let her take the juice of cardus, and if she vomiteth it up, it is a sign of conception. Cast a clean needle into the woman's urine, put it into a bason, let it stand all night, and in the morning if it be coloured with red spots she hath conceived, but if black or rusty, she hath not.

Signs taken from the sex, to shew whether it be male or female. Being with child of a male the right breast swells first, the right eye is more lively than the left, her face well coloured, because such as the blood is, such is the colour ; and the male is conceived in purer blood, and more perfect seed than the female ; red motes in the urine settling down the sediments, foretell that a male is conceived, but if they be white a female. Put the woman's urine which is with child into a glass bottle, let it stand close stopped three days, then strain it through line cloth, and you will find little living creatures. If they be red it is a male, if white it is a female.—To conclude, the most certain sign to give credit unto, is the motion of the infant, for the male moves in the third month, and females in the fourth.

K

CHAP. XIII.

Of untimely births.

WHEN the fruit of the womb comes forth
before the seventh month (that is before
it comes to maturity) it is said to be abortive, and
in effect the children prove abortive (I mean not
alive) if it be born in the eighth month. And
why children born in the seventh or ninth month
may live, and not in the eighth month may seem
strange yet it is true; the cause thereof by some
is ascribed unto the planet under which the child
is born; for every month from the conception to
the birth, is governed by his proper planet. And
in the eighth month Saturn doth predominate,
which is cold and dry: Coldness being an utter
enemy to life, destroys the nature of the child.
Hippocrates gives a better reason, viz. The infant
being every way perfect and complete in the seventh month, desires more air and nutriment than
it had before; which, because he cannot obtain,
the labours for a passage to get out; and if his
spirits become weak and faint and have no
strength sufficient to break the membranes and
come forth as is decreed by nature, that he should
continue in the womb till the ninth month, that
in that time his wearied spirits might again be
strengthened and refreshed: but if he returns to
strive again the eighth month, and be born, he
cannot live, because the day of his birth is either
past or to come. For in the eighth month (saith
Aven) he is weak and infirm; and therefore being
cast into the cold air, his spirits cannot be supported.

Cause.] Untimely birth may be caused by

cold, for as it maketh the fruit of the tree to wither and to fall down before it be ripe, so doth it nip the fruit of the womb before it comes to full perfection, and makes it to be abortive; sometimes by humidity, weakening the faculty that the fruit cannot be restrained till the due time. By dryness or emptiness, defrauding the child of its nourishment. By one of these alvine fluxes of phlebotomy and other evacuations: by inflammations of the womb and other sharp diseases.— Sometimes it is caused by joy, laughter, anger, and especially fear; for in that the heat forsakes the womb, and runs to the heart for help there, so the cold strikes in the matrix, whereby the ligaments are relaxed, and so abortion follows; wherefore, Plato, in his time, commanded that the women should shun all temptation of immoderate joy and grief. Abortion also may be caused by the corruption of the air, by filthy odours, and especially by the smell of the snuff of a candle; also by falls, blows, violent exercise, leaping, dancing, etc.

Signs.] Signs of future abortion are extenuation of the breasts, with a flux of watery milk, pain in the womb, heaviness in the head, unusual weariness in the hips and thys, flowing of the courses. Signs foretelling the fruit to be dead in the womb, are hollowness of the eyes, pain in the head, anguish, horrors, paleness of the face and lips, gnawing of the stomach, no motion of the infant, coldness and looseness of the mouth of the womb, and thickness of the belly, which was above is fallen down, watery and bloody excrements come from the matrix.

CHAP. XIV.

Directions for Breeding Woman.

THE prevention of untimely birth consists in taking away the aforementioned causes which must be effected before and after the conception.

Before the conception, if the body be over hot, cold, dry, or moist, correct it with the contraries; if cacochimical, purge it; if plethriocal, open the liver vein; if too gross extenuate it; if too lean, corroborate and nourish it. All diseases of the womb must be removed as I have shewen.

After conception the air must be temperate, sleep not over much, avoid watching, exercise of body, passions of the mind, loud clamours, and filthy smells; sweet odours are also to be rejected of those that are hysterical. Abstain from all things that provoke either the urine or courses, also from salt, sharp and windy meats; a moderate diet should be observed.

The cough is another accident which accompanieth breeding women, and puts them in great danger of miscarrying, by a continual distillation falling from the brain. To prevent which, shave away the hair from the cornal and satical coissures, and apply thereon this plaister. Take resinæ half an ounce; laudanim one dram; stirachis liquidæ and ficcæ sufficient quantity; dissolve the gums in vinegar, and make a plaister at night going to bed, let her take the fume of these trochisks cast upon the coals.

In breeding woman there is a corrupted matter generated, which flowing to the ventricle, dejecteth the appetite, and causeth vomiting. And the stomach being weak, not able to digest this matter, sometimes sends it to the guts, whereby is caused a flux in the belly, which greatly stirreth up the faculty of the womb. To prevent all these dangers, the stomach must be corroborated as follows: Take lign aloes, nutmeg of each one dram; mace, clove, laudanum, of each two scruples, oil of spik an ounce; musk two grains; oil of mastic, quinces, wormwood, of each half an ounce: make an unguen: for the stomach, to be applied before meals. Another accident which perplexeth a woman with child is sweling of the legs, which happens the first three months by superfluous humours falling down from the stomach and liver; for the cure whereof, take oil of roses two drams; salt vinegar, of each one dram; snake them together until the salt be dissolved, and anoint the legs hot therewith, chaffing it with the hand: By pursuing it more properly, if it may be done without danger, as it may be in the fourth, fifth, or sixth month of purgation; for the child in the womb is compared to an apple on the tree: the first three months it is weak and tender, subject with the apple, to fall away; but afterwards the membranes being strengthened, the fruit remains firmly fastened to the womb, not apt to mischances, and so continues all the seventh Month, till growing nearer the time of its maturity the lagaments are again relaxed (like an apple that is almost ripe) and grows looser every day until the fixed time of delivery. If, therefore, the body is in real need of purging, she may do it without danger, in the fourth, fifth or sixth month, but not before nor after, unless in some sharp diseases. in which the mother and child both are like to perish.

Apply it to the reins in the winter time and remove it every twenty-four hours, lest the reins be ever hot therewith. In the interim anoint the privities and reins with unguent, consitis *æ*; but if it be summet time, and the reins be hot, this plaister following is more proper: Take of red roses one lb. mastick, red sanders, of each two drams pomegrant peel, prepared coriander, of each two drams and an half; barberies two scruples; oil of mastick and quinces, of each one oz. ; juice of plaintain two drams; with pitch make a plaister; anoint the reins also with unguentum sandal.

CHAP. XV.

Directions to be observed by Woman at the Time of their falling in Labour, in order to their safe Delivery, with Directions for midwives.

AND thus having given necessary directions for child-bearing woman, how to govern themselves during the time of their pregnacy, I shall add what is necessary for them to observe, in order to their delivery,

The time of birth drawing near let the woman send for a skillful midwife, and that rather too soon than too late ; and against which time let her prepare a pallet, bed, or conch near the fire, that the midwife and her assistants may pass round and help on every side, as occasion requires, having a change of linen ready, and a small stool to rest her feet

against, she having more force when they are bowed, then when they are otherwise.

Having thus provided, when the woman feels
her pain come, and weather not cold, let her walk
about the room, resting herself by turns upon the
bed, and so expect the coming down of her water, which is a humour contracted in one of the outward membranes and flows thence when it is broken by the strugling of the child, their being no
direct time fixed for the efflux, though generally
it flows not above two hours before the birth; motion will likewise cause the womb to open and dilate itself, when lying long in bed will be uneasy;
yet, if she be very weak, she may take some gentle cordial to refresh herself, if her pain will
permit.

If her travail be tedious, she may revive her
spirits with taking chicken or nutton-broth, or she
may take a poached fig, but must take heed of eating to excess.

As for the postures woman are delivered in, they
are many, some lying in their bed, sitting in
their bed, or chair; some, again, on their knees,
being supported upon their arms; but the most safe
and commodious way is in the bed, and then the
midwife ought to mind the following rules.—Let
her lay the woman upon her back, her head a little
raised by the help of a pillow, having the like help
to support her reins and buttocks, and that her rump
may lie high, for if she lies low, she cannot be well
delivered. Let her keep her knees and thighs as
far distance as she can, her legs bowed together and
her buttocks, the soals of her feet and heels being
placed on a little log of timber, placed for that purpose, that she may strain the stronger; And then,

to facilitate it, let a woman stroke or press the upper part of the belly gently, and by degrees :   Nor
must the woman herself be faint-hearted, but of good
courage, forcing herself by straining and holding
her breath.

In case of delivery, the midwife must wait with
patience till the child, or other members, burst the
membrane ; for, if, thro' ignorance, or haste to go to
other women, as some have done, the midwife tears
the membrane with her nails, she endangers both
the woman and the child ; for, its laying dry, and
wanting that slipperiness that should make it easy,
it comes forth with great pain.

Where the head appears, the midwife must gently hold it between her hands, and draw the child at
such times as the woman's pains are upon her, & at
no other ; slipping by degrees her fore-fingers under
his arm-pits, not using a rough hand in drawing it
forth, lets by that means, the tender infant receive
any deformity of body. As soon as the child is tak-
en forth, which is, for the most part, with its face
downward, let it be laid on its back, that it may more
freely receive external respiration ; then cut the
navelstring, about three inches from the body, ty-
ing that end which adheres to the belly with a silk-
en string, as near as you can ; then cover the head
and stomach of the child well, suffering nothing
to come upon the face.

The child being thus brought forth, and, if,
healthy, lay it by, and let the midwife regard the
patient in drawing forth the secundines ; and this
she may do by wagging and stiring them up and
down, and afterwards, with a gentle hand, drawing
them forth : And, if the work be difficult, let the
woman hold salt in her hands, and thereby she will

know whether the membranes be broke or not. It may be also known by causing her to strain or vomit, by putting a finger down her throat, or by straining or moving her lower parts, but let all be done out of hand. If this fail, let her take a draught of raw elder-water, 'or yolk of a new-laid egg, and smell to a piece of assafœtida, especially if she be troubled with a windy cholic. If she happen to take cold, it is a great obstruction to the coming down of the secundines; and in such cases, the women ought to chaff the woman's belly gently, not only to break the wind, but oblige the fecundines to com • down. But these proving ineffectual, the midwife must chatter with her hand the extern or orifice of the womb, and gently draw it forth.

CHAP. XVI.

In Cases of Extremity, what ought to be observed, especially to Women, who, in their Travail, are attended with a flux of Blood, Convulsions, and Fits of the Wind.

IF the woman's labour be hard and difficult, greater regard must then be had, than at other times; and first of all, the situation of the womb, and posture of lying, must be across the bed, being held by strong persons, to prevent her slipping down or moving herself in the operation of the surgeon; Her thighs must be put asunder, as far distant as may be, and so held; whilst her head must lean upon a bolster, and the reins of her back supported after the same manner; her rump and buttocks being lifted up, observing to cover her stomach, belly and thighs with warm linen, to keep them from the cold.

The woman being in this posture, let the operator put up his hand, if he find the neck of the womb dilated, and remove the contracted blood that obstructs the passage of the birth ; and having, by degrees, gently made way, let him tenderly move the infant, his hand being first anointed with sweet butter, or a harmless pomatum. And if the waters be not come down, then, without difficulty, may they be let forth : when, if the infant should attempt to break out with its head foremost, or cross, he may gently turn it to find the feet ; which having done, let him draw forth the one and fasten it to a ribbon, then put it up again, and by degrees find the other, bringing them as close and even as may be, and between whiles, let the woman breathe, urging her to strain to help nature to perfect the birth, that he may draw it forth ; and the readier to do it, that his hold may be the surer, he must wrap a linen cloth about the child's thighs, observing to bring it into the world with its face downwards.

In case of a flux of blood, if the neck of the womb be open, it must be considered whether the infant or secundine comes first, which the latter sometimes happening to do, stops the mouth of the womb and hinders the birth, endangering both the woman and the child ; but, in this case, the secundines must be removed by a swift turn ; and indeed they have by their so coming down deceived many, who feeling their softness, supposed the womb was not dilated; and by this means the woman and the child, or at least the latter, has been lost. The secundines moved, the child must be sought for, and drawn forth, as has been directed ; and if in such a case the woman or child die, the midwife or surgeon is blameless, because they did their true endeavour.

If it appears, upon enquiry, that the secundines come first, let the woman be delivered with all convenient expedition, because a great flux of blood will follow, for the veins are opened, and upon this account two things are to be considered:

First, The manner of the secundines advancing, whether it be much or little; if the former, and the head of the child appear first. it may be guided and directed towards the neck of the womb, as in the case of natural birth; but, if there appear any difficulty in the delivery, the best way is to search for the feet. and thereby draw it forth; but if the latter, the secundine may be put back with a gentle hand, and the child first taken forth.

But, if the secundine be far advanced, so that it cannot be put back, and the child follow it close, then are the secundines to be taken forth with much care, as swift as may be, and laid without cutting the entrail that is fastened to them, for thereby you may be guided to the infant, which, whether alive or dead, must be drawn forth by the feet, in all haste, though it is not to be acted unless in any great necessity, for in other cases the secundines ought to come last.

And in drawing forth a dead child, let these directions be carefully observed by the surgeon, viz. if the child be found dead, its head foremost delivery will be the more difficult; for it is an apparent sign the woman's strength begins to fail her, and that the child being dead, and wanting its natural force, can be no ways assisting to its delivery, wherefore the most certain and safe way for the surgeon is, to put up his left hand, sliding it as hollow in the palm as he can, into the neck of the womb, and into the lower part thereof towards the feet, and then between the head of the infant and the neck of the matrix, when having a hook in the right hand, couch it close and slip it above the left hand, between the head of the child and the flat of the hand, fixing it in the bars of the temple towards the eye ; for want of a convenient coming at these in the occiputal-bone, observe still to the left hand in its place and with it gently moving and stirring the head ; and so, with the right hand and hook, draw the child forward, admonishing the woman to put forth her utmost strength; still drawing when the woman's pangs are upon her ; the head being drawn out, with all speed, he must slip his hand up under the arm-holes of the child, and take it quite out, giving these things to the woman—A toast of fine wheaten bread in a quarter of an ounce of ipocras wine.

If it so happen that any inflammation, swelling, or congealed blood be contracted in the matrix, under the film of these tumours, either before or after the birth, where the matter appears thinner, then let the midwife, with a pen-knife or an incision instrument, launch it, and press out the corruption, healing it with a pessary dipped in oil of red roses.

If at any time, through cold, or some violence, the child happen to be swelled in any part, or hath contracted a watery humour, if it remain alive, such means must be used as are least injurious to the child and the mother; but if it be dead, that humour must be let out by incision, to facilitate the birth.

If (as it often happens) that the child comes
with its feet foremost, and the hands dilating
themselves from the hips; in such cases, the midwife must be prepared with necessary ointment,
to stroke and anoint the infant with, to help its
coming forth, lest it turn again into the womb,
holding at the same time, both the arms of the infant close to the hips, that so it may issue forth
after its manner; but if it proves too big, the
womb must be well anointed.   The woman may
also take sneezing-powder, to make her strain :
Those who attend may gently stroke her belly, to
make the birth descend, and keep the birth from
retiring back.

And sometimes it falls out that the child coming
with the feet foremost, has its arms extended
above its head ; but the midwife must not receive
it so, but put it back again into the womb, unless
the passage be extraordinary wide, and then she
must anoint the child and the womb ; nor is it
safe to draw it forth, which may be done in this
manner—the woman must lie on her back, with
her head depressed, and her buttocks raised ; and
the midwife, with a gentle hand, must compress
the belly of the woman towards the midwife, by
that means to put back the infant, observing to
turn the face of the child towards the back of its
mother, raising up its thighs and buttocks towards
her navel, that so the birth may be more natural.

If a child happens to come forth with one foot,
the arm being extended along the side, and the
other foot turned backward, then must the woman
be instantly brought to her bed, and laid in the
posture above described, at which time the midwife must carefully put back the foot so appearing,

and the woman rocking herself from one side to the other, till she find the child is turned, but must not alter her posture, nor turn upon her face. After which she may expect her pains, and must have great assistance and cordials to revive and support her spirits.

At other times it happens that the child lies across in the womb, and falls upon its side; in this case the woman must not be urged in her labour, neither can any expect the birth in such a manner —therefore the midwife, when she finds it so, must use great diligence to reduce it to its right form, or at least to such a form in the womb, as may make the delivery possible and more easy, by moving the buttocks, and guiding the head to the passage; and if she be successful herein, let her again try by rocking herself to and fro, and wait with patience till it alters its manner of lying.

Sometimes the child hastens the birth, by expanding its legs and arms; in which as in the former the woman must rock herself, but not with violence, till she finds those parts fall to their proper stations, or it may be done by a gentle compression of the womb, but if neither of them prevail, the midwife with her hand must close the legs of the infant, and if she come at them, do the like to the arms, and so draw it forth; but if it can be reduced of itself, to the posture of a natural birth, it is better.

If the infant comes forward with both knees foremost and the hands hanging down upon the thighs, then must the midwife put both knees upward, till the feet appear; taking hold of which with her left hand, let her keep her right hand on the side of the child, and in that posture endeavour to bring it forth.

But if she cannot do this, then also must the woman rock herself till the child is in a convenient posture for delivery.

Sometimes it happens, that the child passes forward with one arm stretched on its thighs, and the other raised over its head, and the feet stretched out length in the womb ; in such a case the midwife must not attempt to receive the child in that posture, but must lay the woman on the bed, in the manner aforesaid, making a soft and gentle compression on her belly, to oblige the child to retire, which if it does not, then must the midwife thrust it back by the shoulder, and bring the arm that was stretched above the head, to its right station ; for there is more danger in these extremities, and therefore the midwife must anoint her hands first, and the womb of the woman with sweet butter, or a proper pomatum, thursting her hand as near as she can, to the arm of the infant, and bring it to the side.

But if this cannot be done, let the woman be laid on her bed to rest awhile, in which time, perhaps the child may be reduced to a better posture, which the midwife finding, she must draw tenderly the arms close to the hips, and so receive it.

If an infant come with its buttocks foremost, and almost double, then the midwife, anointing her hand must thrust it up, and greatly heaving up the buttocks and back, strive to turn the head to the passage, but not too hastily, lest the infant's retiring should shape it worse, and therefore it cannot be turned with the hand, the woman must rock herself on the bed, taking some comfortable things as may support her spirits, till she perceives the child to turn.

If the child's neck be bowed; and it comes forward with its shoulders, as sometimes it doth, with the hand and feet streached upwards; the midwife must gently move the shoulders, that she may direct the head to the passage ; and the better to effect it, the woman must rock herself as afforesaid.

These, and other the like methods are to be observed, in case a woman hath twins, or three children at a birth as sometimes happens. For as the single birth hath but one natural way, and many unnatural forms, even so it may be in double or treple births.

Wherefore, in all such cases, the midwife must take care to receive that first which is nearest the passage, but not letting the other go, lest by retiring it should change the form. And when one is born, she must be speedy in bringing forth the other—and this birth, if it be in the natural way, is more easy, because the children are commonly less than those of a single birth, and so require a lesser passage. But if this birth come unnaturally, it is far more dangerous than the other.

In the birth of twins, let the midwife be very careful that the secundines be naturally brought forth, lest the womb being delivered of its burthen fall and, and so the secundines continue longer than is consistant with the woman's safety.

But if one of the twins happen to come with the head, and the other with the feet foremost, then let the midwife deliver the natural birth first, and if she cannot turn the other out, draw it out in the posture it presseth forward, but if that with its feet downward be foremost, she may deliver that first turning the other side.

But in this case, the midwife must carefully see that it be not a monstrous birth, instead of twins a body with two heads, or two bodys joined together, which you may soon see; if both the heads come foremost by putting up her hand between them as high as she can, and then if she find they are twins, she may gently put one of them asside to make way for the other, taking the first which is most advanced, having the other, that she do not change its situation.

And for the safety of the first child, as soon as it comes forth out of the womb, the midwife must tie the navel-string as has been before directed, and also bind it with a large and long fillet. that part of the navel that is fastened to the secundies the more ready to find them.

The second infant being born, let the midwife carefully examine weather their be not two secundines, for sometimes it falls out, that by the shortness of the ligaments, it retires back to the prejudice of the woman.   Wherefore lest the womb should close, it is most expedient to hasten them forth with all convenient speed.

If two infants are joined together by the body as sometimes it monstrously falls out, then though the heads should come foremost, yet it is convenient if possible to turn them, and draw them forth by the feet, observing that when they come to the hips to draw them out as soon as may be.

And here great care ought to be used in anointing and widening the passage. But these sort of birth rarely happen.

L 2

CHAP. XVII.

How Child-bearing Woman are ordered after De-

livery.

IF a woman has had very hard labour, it is ne-cessary she should be rapped up in sheep's skin taken off before it is cold, applying the fleshy side to her reins and belly. Or, for want of this the skin of a hare, or coney, flead off as soon as killed, may be applyed to the same parts·

Let the woman afterwards be swathed with fine linen cloth, about a quarter of a yard in breadth, chafling her belly before it is swathed with oil of St. John's wort; after that raize up the matrix with a linen cloth many times folded, then with a little pillow, or quilt over her flanks, and place the swathe somewhat above the haunches, wind-ing it pretty stiff, apply at the same time a warm cloth to her nipples, and not presently applying the remedies to keep back the milk, by reason of the body at such a time is out of fraim, for, there is neither vein nor artery which does not strong-ly bent and remedies to drive back the milk being of a dissolving nature, it is improper to apply them to the breasts during such disorder, lest by to doing evil humours be contracted in the breasts Wherefore twelve hours at least ought to be al-lowed for the circulation and settlement of the-blood, and what was cast upon the lungs, by the vehemant agitation during the labour, to retire to its proper recepticles.

She must by no means sleep presently after de-livery, but about four hours after she may take broth caudle, or such liquod victuals as are nour-ishing; and if she is disposed to sleep, she may

be very eafely permitted   And this is as much
(in case of a natural birth) as ought immediately
to be done.

If the mother intend to nurse her child now
she may take something more than ordinary,
to increase the milk by degrees, which must be of
no continuance, but drawn by the child otherwise.
— In this case likewise obferv, to let her have cor-
riander or fennel-seed, boiled in her barley broth,
and if no feveer trouble her' she may drink now
and then a small quantity of white wine or claret.

And after the fear of a fever or contradiction of
humour in the breasts is over, she may be nourished more plentifully with the broth of pullets or
veal, &c. which must not be till after eight days
from the time of her delivery, at which time the
womb unless some accident hinder, hath purged
itself,   It then be expected to give cold meat, but
let it be spareing that so she may the better
gather strength.

And let her, during the time, rest quietly and
free from disturbance, not sleeping in the day
time if she can avoid it.

C H A P. XVII.

How to expell the Chotic from Women in Child-birth.

THESE pains frequently afflict the women
no less than in pains of her labour, and are by
the ignorant taken many times the one for the
other, and sometimes they happen both at the
same instant, which is occasioned by a raw crude
and watery matter in the stomach, contracted

through ill digestion, and while such pain continues the woman's travail is retarded.

Therefore, to expell such fits of the cholic, take two ounces of oil of sweet almonds, and an onuce of cinnamond water, with three or four drops of spirit of ginger, then let the woman drink it off.

If the pain prove the griping of the guts, and long after delivery, then take the root of a great comfery, one dram, nutmeg and peach kernels, of each two scruples, and give them to the woman as she is laid down, in two or three spoonfuls of white wine ; but if she be feverish, then let it be in as much of warm broth.

THE

FAMILY PHYSICIAN.

BEING CHOICE AND APPROVED REMEDIES FOR SEVERAL DISTEMPERS INCIDENT TO HU-MAN BODIES, &C.

FAMILY PHYSICIAN.

Being choice and approved remedies for several distempers incident to human bodies, &c.

For Apoplexy

TAKE man's-skul prepared, powder of the root of male-prony, of each an ounce and a half; contrayera, bastard dittany, angelica, zedoary, of each two drams, mix and make a powder, whereof you may take half a dram, or a dram.

A Powder for the Epilepsy or Falling Sickness.

Take of opoponax, crude antimony, dragon's-blood, castor penny-seeds, of each an equal quantity, make a subtile powder. The dose, from half a dram in black-cherry-water. Before you take it the stomach must be cleansed with some proper vomit, as that of Mysinct's emetic tarter, from four grains to six. If for children, salts of vitriol, from a scruple to half a dram.

A Vomit for Swimming in the Head

Take cream of tarter half a scruple, castor two grains, mix all together for a vomit, to be taken at four o'clock in the afternoon. At night, going to bed, it will be very proper to take a dose of apostolic powder.

For an Head-Ach of long Standing.

Take the juice of powder, or distilled water of hog-lice, and continue the use of it.

For Spitting of Blood.

Take conserve of comfrey, and of hipps, of each an ounce and an half; conserve of red roses three ounces, dragon's-blood a dram, species of hyscinths two scruples, red coral a dram, mix, and with syrup of red poppies make a soft electuary. Take the quantity of a walnut night and morning.

A Powder against Vomitting.

Take crabs' eyes, red coral, each ivory, of each two drams, burnt; hartshorn one dram cinnamon and red sanders of each one dram make a full subtile powder, and take half a dram.

For a Looseness.

Take of Venice treacle and diascordinm, of each half a dram, in warm ale, water-gruel, or what you bestlike, last at night going to bed.

For the Bloody-Flux.

Eirst, take a dram of the powder of rhubarb in a sufficient quantity of the conserve of red roses, early in the morning; then, at night, take of fortified or roasted rhubarb half a dram, diascordium a dram and a half, liquid laudanum cydoniated a scruple; mix and make a bolus.

For Inflammation in the Lungs.

Take curious water ten ounces, water of red poppies three ounces, syrup of poppies an ounce, pearl prepared a dram, make a julip, and take six spoonfulls every fourth hour.

Pills very profitable in an Asthma.

Take gum ammoniac and bedellium, dissolved in

vinegar of squills, of each half an ounce ; powder of the leaves of hedge, mustard and savoury, of each half a dram. flour of sulphur three drams, and with sufficient quantity of syrup of sulphur, make a mass of small pills, three whereof take every morning.

An Electuary for the dropsy.

Take choice rhubarb one dram, gum lac prepared two drams, zyloaloes, cinnamon, long birthwort of each half an ounce, the best English saffron half a scruple, with syrup of chycory and rhubarb make an electuary. Take the quantity of a nutmeg, or a walnut every morning fasting.

For Weakness in Woman.

After a gentle purge ot two, take the following decoction, viz. A quantity of a pound of lignum vitæ. sassafras two ounces raisins of the sun eight ounces, liquorice sliced two ounces; boil all in six quarts of water to a gallon, strain and keep it for use. Take half a pint at four o'clock in the after-noon, the third last at night going to bed.

A Clyster proper in a Pleurisy.

Take clean Faench barley an handful, leaves of mallows, mercury, violets, of each a handful and a half, twelve damask prunes boil all in a sufficient quantity of water to a pint and a half; when strained, add an ounce and a half of fresh cassa and red sugar, with the yolk of an egg. This may be injected every other day.

An Ointment for the same

Take the oil of violets, sweet almonds, of each an ounce, with whey and a little saffron make an

M

ointment; warm it, and bathe with it the part affected.

An Ointment for the Itch.

Take sulphur vive in powder half an ounce, oil
of tartar per dilinquim a sufficient quantity, ointment of roses four ounces, make a liniment; to
which add a scruple of the oil of rhodium to aro-
matise it, and rub the part affected with it.

For a running Scab.

Take two pounds of tar, incorporate into a thick
mass with good sifted ashes, boil the mass in fountain water, adding leaves of ground-ivy, white hore-
hound, fumitory, roots of sharp-pointed dock, and
of elecampane, of each four handfuls; make a
bath to be used, with care of taking cold.

For Worms in Children.

Take worm-seed half a-dram, flour of sulphur
a dram, sal prunelle half a dram, mix and make a
powder. Give as much as will lie on a silver three-
pence, night or morning, in treacle or honey. Or
for people grown up, you may add a sufficient quantity of aloe rosatum, and so make them up into pills,
three or four thereof may be taken every morning.

For the Gripes in Children.

Give a drop or two of the oil of anniseeds in a
spoonful of panada, milk, or what else you think fit.

*Of the Judgment of Physiognomy taken from all
Parts of the Human Body.*

HE whose hair is partly curled and partly
hanging down, is commonly a wise man or a
fool; or else as very knave as he is a fool. He
whose hair groweth thick on his temples and his
brows, is by nature simple, vain, luxurious, lustful, credulous, clownish in his speech and conversation. He whose hair is of a reddish complexion
is, for the most part, proud, deceitful, detracting,
venerous, and full of envy. He whose hair is very fair, is, for the most part, a man fit for all praise-
worthy actions, a lover of honours, and more inclined to good than evil; careful to perform whatsoever is committed to his care; secret in carrying on any business, and fortunate. Hair of a yellowish colour, shews a man to be good, and will-
ing to do any thing, fearful, bashful, weak of body,
but strong in the abilities of his mind, and more
apt to remember than to revenge an injury. He
whose hair turns grey or hoary in the time of his
youth, is generally given to women, vain, false, un-
stable and talkative.—*Note*, That whatsoever sig-
nification the hair has in men, it is the same in
women also.

As whose forehead riseth in a round, signifies a
man liberal, of a good understanding, inclined to
virtue. He whose forehead is very low and little,
is of a good understanding, magnanimous, but extremely bold and confident, and a pretender to
love and honour. He whose forehead seems
sharp and pointed up in the corners of his temples,
is a man naturally vain, fickle and weak in intellectuals.—Ne whose brow is full of wrinkles, and

hath, as it were, a coming down in the middle of his forehead, is one of a great spirit, a great wit, void of deceit, and yet of a hard fortune. He whose forehead is long and high, and jutting forth, is honest, but weak and simple, and of an hard fortune.

Those eye-brows that are much arched, whether in man or woman, and which by a frequent motion, elevate themselves, shew the person to be proud, high-spirited, vain-glorious, a lover of beauty, and indifferently inclined to their good or evil.—He whose eye-brows are thick, and have but little hair upon them, is weak in his intellectuals, and too credulous.

Great and full eyes, either in man or woman, shew the person to be, for the most part, slothful, bold, envious, a bad concealer of secrets, miserable, vain, given to lying, and yet of a bad memory, slow of invention, weak of his intellectuals, and yet very much conceited of that little wisdom he thinks himself master of. He whose eyes are hollow in his head, and therefore discerns well at a great distance, is one that is suspicious, proud and treacherous; but he whose eyes are as it were, starting out of his head, is a simple foolish person. He who stands studiously and acutely, with his eyes and eye-lids downward, it denotes him to be malicious impious towards God, and false towards men. Those whose eyes is always a twinkling, and which move backward and forward, shews the person to be luxurious and unfaithful. If a person has any superstition. They who have eyes like oxen, are persons of a good nutriment but of a week memory, and of a dull understanding ; but those whose eyes are neither two little nor two big, and inclining to black, do signify a man mild, peacible. honest, witty, and of a good understanding, and one that when need requires will be servisible to his friend.

A long and thin nose, denots a man bold, curious and vain, weak and credulous. A long nose, the tip bending down, shews the person to be wise and discreat. A bottle nose denote a man to be impettuous in obtaining his desires. He who has a long and large nose, is an admirer of the fair sex, and well accomplished for the wars of Venus, but ignorant of any thing else. A nose very round at. the end of it, having but little nostrils, shews the person to be very munificent and liberal, true to his trust, but very proud, credulous and vain. He whose nose is more red than any other part of his face, is thereby denoted to be covetous. A thick nose with wide nostrils, denotes a man dull of apprehension, simple, and a liar.

When the nostrils are close and thin, they denote a man to have but little testicles, and to be very desirous of the enjoyment of women, but modest in his conversation ; but he whose nostrils are great and wide, is usually well hung and lustful, but withal of an envious, bold and treacherous disposition, and though dull of understanding yet confident enough.

A great and wide mouth, shews the man to be bold, warlike, shameless, and stout, a great liar, and a great talker and carrier of news, and also a great eater, but as for his intellectuals they are very dull.

M 2

The lips, when they are very big and blabber-ing, shew a person to be credulous, foolish, dull and stupid, aud apt to be inticed to any thing.

When the teeth are small, but weak in perform-ing their office, and especially if they are short and few, though they shew the party to be of a weak constitution, yet they denote him to be of no ex-traordinary understanding, and not only so, but also of a meek disposition, honest, faithful and se-cret in whatever they are trusted with.

A tongue too swift in speech, shews a man to be very foolish and vain. A stammering tongue signifies a weak understanding, and a wavering mind. A very thick and rough tongue, denotes a man to be apprehensive, full of compliments, yet treacherous and prone to impiety.

A faint voice, attended with little breath, shews a person to be of good uuderstanding but timerous.

A thick full chin, abounding with peace, honest and true to his trust. A picked chin shews one to be of a lofty spirit.

Yong men's beards usually begin to grow on their chins at fifteen years of age, and sooner; these hairs proceed from the superfluity of heat, the fumes whereof ascend to the chin and cheeks, like smoke to the funnel of a chimney ; there are few women that have hair on their chins, and the reason is, those humours which cause hair to grow on men's cheeks, are evacuated by women, in their monthly courses.

Great thick ears are certain signs of a foolish person, of a bad memory, and worse understand-ing ; but small and thin cars shews a person to be of good wit and understanding, grave, secret, thrif-ty, modest, of a good memory, & williug to oblige.

A face apt to sweat on every occasion, shews the person to be of a hot constitution, vain and luxurious, of a good stomach, but of a bad understanding, and worse conversation. A lean face shews a man to be both bold in speech and action, but withal foolish and deceitful. A face every way of due proportion, denotes an ingenuous person, one fit for any thing, and much inclined to what is good.

General observations, worthy of Note.

WHEN you find a red man to be faithful, a a tall man to be wise, a fat man to be swift on foot, a lean man to be a fool, a handsome man to be proud, a poor man not to be envious, a knave to be no liar, an upright man not too bold and harty to his own loss ; one that drawls when he speaks, not to be crafty and circumventing ; one that winks on another with his eyes, not to be false and deceitful —a sailor and a hangman, to be pitiful, a poor man to build churches, a quack doctor to have a good conscience, a bailiff not to be a merciless villain, an hostess not to over-reckon you, and an usurer to be charitable : Then say you have found a progidy, and men acting contrary to the common course of nature.

FINIS.

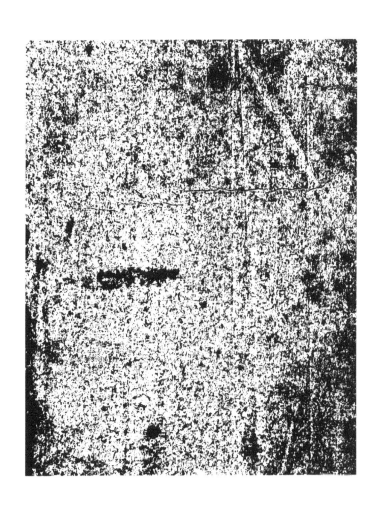